LESSONS IN EKG INTERPRETATION
A BASIC SELF-INSTRUCTIONAL GUIDE
Second Edition

Charles P. Summerall III, M.D.
Associate Professor
Department of Medicine
Medical University of South Carolina College of Medicine
Cardiologist
Veterans Administration Medical Center
Charleston, South Carolina

Churchill Livingstone
New York, Edinburgh, London, Melbourne, Tokyo

Library of Congress Cataloging-in-Publication Data
Summerall, Charles P.
    Lessons in EKG interpretation : a basic self-instructional guide /
Charles P. Summerall III. — 2nd ed.
        p. cm.
    Includes index.
    ISBN 0-443-08778-4
    1. Electrocardiography—Programmed instruction. 2. Heart-
-Diseases—Diagnosis—Programmed instruction. I. Title.
    [DNLM: 1. Electrocardiography—programmed instruction. 2. Heart
Diseases—diagnosis—programmed instruction. WG 18 S957L]
    RC683.5.E5S83 1991
    616.1'207547'077—dc20
    DNLM/DLC
    for Library of Congress   91-200
                                                                              CIP

The following figures have been reprinted with permission from Charles P.
Summerall, J. Mangiaracina, and Jan McNeely : *Monitoring Heart Rhythm,*
2nd Edition. Copyright © 1982 by John Wiley & Sons: 1.1; 24.8; 25.2; 25.10;
26.1 to 26.7.

Distributed in the United Kingdom by Churchill Livingstone, Robert
Stevenson House, 1–3 Baxter's Place, Leith Walk, Edinburgh EH1 3AF, and
by associated companies, branches, and representatives throughout the
world.

Acquisitions Editor: *Avé McCracken*
Copy Editor: *Christina Joslin*
Production Designer: *Patricia McFadden*
Production Supervisor: *Christina Hippeli*

Printed in the United States of America

First published in 1991   7 6 5 4 3 2 1

LESSONS IN EKG INTERPRETATION
A BASIC SELF-INSTRUCTIONAL GUIDE

Second Edition

ll Ltd., London, N.21 Cat. No. 1207   DG 02242/71

Preface to the Second Edition

This new edition, based on a long experience with medical students and housestaff in a hospital EKG station, continues to emphasize a self-instructional approach to fundamental aspects of clinical EKG analysis. The text has been streamlined and abbreviated wherever possible. Additional material concerns principles of the signal-averaged EKG and of probability concepts related to EKG interpretation.

As the knowledge explosion in medical science pursues its exponential path, this textbook hopes to offer a sound and relatively rapid mastery of a skill that remains an essential component of daily patient care.

Charles P. Summerall III, M.D.

Preface to the First Edition

This textbook is especially designed for medical students who are beginning to use electrocardiograms (EKGs) clinically. The self-instruction method employed may also be useful for physicians in residency training, for experienced intensive-care nurses, and for others who wish to review or expand basic skills in EKG interpretation.

Medical students are not in an enviable position as they first undertake EKG analysis in a clinical setting. Typically, previous courses have given them some understanding of cardiac anatomy and cellular electrophysiology, but the language of electrocardiography is only vaguely familiar to them. Even more important, they have little grasp of the limitations of this diagnostic method. As they first encounter patients with chest pain, hypertension, or heart rhythm disorders, their opportunities to learn about EKG abnormalities are fragmentary.

Lessons in EKG Interpretation employs a simple self-instruction design that leads to mastery of a difficult vocabulary and of basic skills through application and repetition. These lessons provide a framework for everday use of the EKG as currently required in every primary care field of medicine. They emphasize practical rather than theoretical issues and highlight common conceptual problems or pitfalls.

Successive advances in diagnostic cardiology have clarified both the validity and limitations of 12-lead EKG interpretation. As for many laboratory methods, knowledge of the individual patient governs the meaning of an abnormal electrocardiographic finding. This knowledge is available to the primary physician, but not to the cardiologist in a hospital EKG station. The skills emphasized in this text are intended to guide the reader toward effective and realistic use of EKGs in his or her personal practice.

I am indebted to Ms. Donna Fender, without whose patient secretarial help this book would not exist, and to Ms. Betty Goodwin, whose skill as a medical illustrator will be evident to all users of this text.

Charles P. Summerall III, M.D.

Contents

Instructions

The sequence of units in this textbook is patterned on the usual sequence of steps in routine EKG interpretation. This sequence first requires identification of abnormal waveforms, an objective analysis that is generally within the capacity of a computer program. The second phase of interpretation is more abstract, requiring inferences based on composite features of the 12-lead EKG and on whatever information is available about the individual patient. Unit 1 concerns the basic features of a normal EKG. Units 2 through 5 describe abnormal patterns of each component of the EKG complex. Unit 6 expands the discussion of rhythm disorders introduced in previous units. In Unit 7, the EKG abnormalities associated with important disease states are brought together.

The textbook uses a self-instructional design based on practice and repetition. Each lesson consists of text segments for study, followed by practice questions or EKGs for interpretation. A review of correct answers follows each practice segment. Practice questions are principally of the sentence completion type. Your response may be flexible to some extent and need not correspond exactly to terms used in the review of correct answers. Major emphasis is on the need to use and think about the vocabulary of electrocardiography. Among different cardiologists or different medical centers, EKG terminology is not well standardized, and there is clearly room for differences of opinion on nomenclature. The Glossary following Unit 7 explains selected terms that are often confusing.

You will need standard EKG calipers to complete practice questions. Because measurement of small EKG intervals is not a precise process, your measurements need not correspond exactly to those given in the text, but should closely approximate them.

1 Characteristics of a Normal EKG

Lesson 1

Events of the Cardiac Cycle

The electrocardiogram (EKG) provides a fascinating but incomplete view of a remarkably consistent and durable phenomenon—the heartbeat. It records a sequence of electrical events that correspond to contraction and relaxation of the heart chambers, but it supplies no direct information about the effectiveness of the heart's pumping action. It also displays only indirectly the function of pacing and conducting tissues, for these highly specialized muscle fibers form relatively small nodes and bundles that do not generate electrical potentials large enough to be recorded from the body surface.

To a large extent, the pacing and conducting system determines the characteristics of the EKG. This system initiates the heartbeat and governs the spread of electrical activity through the atria and ventricles. Lesson 1 concerns the normal anatomy of the pacing and conducting tissues, their basic normal physiology, and their relation to the electrical and hemodynamic events of the heart cycle.

LOCATION AND DIMENSIONS OF PACING AND CONDUCTING TISSUES

Electrical activity of the normal heart cycle begins in the *sinoatrial (SA) node* located in the anterolateral wall of the right atrium near the entrance of the superior vena cava. The node is approximately cylindrical, about 10 mm long and 2 mm wide. Electrical activity spreads from the SA node to muscle fibers throughout the atria and to the *atrioventricular (AV) node,* flowing preferentially through three conduction pathways, the internodal tracts.

The AV node lies in the inferior portion of the right atrium near the center of the heart where the walls of the four heart chambers meet. It is a flattened structure about 1 mm thick and 7 mm × 4 mm in its major dimensions.

Complete the following sentences:

1. Both the _____ node and the _____ node are located in the wall of the _____ atrium.

2. At the onset of the cardiac cycle, electrical activity spreads from the _____ node to the right and left _____ and to the _____ node, spreading preferentially through the _____ tracts.

3. In Figure 1-1, line A indicates the _____ ; line B indicates the _____ ; line C indicates the _____ .

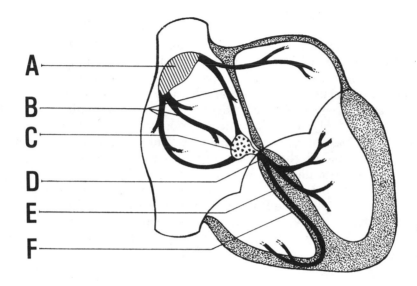

Figure 1-1   Principal structures of cardiac pacing and conduction system.

Review.   The sinoatrial (SA) node, A in Figure 1-1, and the atrioventricular (AV) node, C in Figure 1-1, lie in the right atrium. Electrical activity from the SA node spreads to the atria and to the AV node through internodal tracts, B in Figure 1-1.

On its ventricular aspect, the AV node joins the *His bundle,* a structure described by Professor Wilhelm His in 1893. This conduction pathway is about 10 mm long and lies at the top of the ventricular septum. The AV node and the His bundle together form the only normal path for the spread of atrial electrical activity to the ventricles. An impulse that enters the ventricle through the His bundle is termed *supraventricular,* originating above the ventricles.

The His bundle divides into two branches that descend on opposite sides of the ventricular septum. The *right bundle branch* (RBB) is a long narrow structure that descends on the right side of the septum toward the right ventricular apex. The *left bundle branch* (LBB) is more complex. It has a compact initial portion less than 1 cm long located at the top of the ventricular septum. It then divides and spreads over the left side of the septum, forming two groups of fibers, the *anterior and posterior fascicles* of the LBB. The bundle branches terminate in an extensive network of *Purkinje fibers* that spreads beneath the endocardium to the entire ventricular muscle mass. Ventricular conduction pathways below the AV node are termed collectively the *His-Purkinje system*.

Complete the following sentences:

1. To reach the ventricles, electrical activity from the right atrium must pass through both the _____ node and the _____ bundle.

2. The _____ bundle branch has a more simple structure than the _____ bundle branch.

3. Both bundle branches lie in close relationship to the sides of the _____ .

4. The _____ bundle branch has an _____ fascicle and a _____ fascicle.

5. In Figure 1-1, line D indicates the _____ bundle; line E indicates the _____ branch; line F indicates the _____ .

Review. The AV node and the His bundle (D in Figure 1-1) form the only normal conduction path to the ventricles from the right atrium. The LBB (E in Figure 1-1) is more complex than the RBB (F in Figure 1-1). It has anterior and posterior fascicles. Both bundle branches are closely related to the ventricular septum.

SPECIAL FUNCTIONS OF THE PACING AND CONDUCTION SYSTEM

In a normal heart, *spontaneous electrical impulse formation,* or automatic pacing, is confined to structures of the pacing and conduction system. Automatic pacing activity may occur in the SA node, in the AV junction at the region where the AV node joins the His bundle, and in ventricular Purkinje fibers. Each structure has an inherent natural rate of impulse formation:

SA node—60 to 100 impulses per minute
AV junction—40 to 50 impulses per minute
Purkinje fibers—35 impulses per minute

The most rapid pacing focus, in the SA node, normally dominates all others. When a focus outside the SA node captures the heart, the impulse is termed *ectopic,* meaning "out-of-place."

A second category of special function concerns the *velocity of impulse conduction* through specialized pathways. This function determines many features of the EKG. The AV node has slow conduction velocity, allowing a delay between atrial activation and ventricular activation. In contrast, the normal His—Purkinje system conducts rapidly, permitting prompt spread of electrical activity throughout the ventricles. Conduction through unspecialized cardiac muscle fibers is slow, but provides an alternate path if His—Purkinje fibers are interrupted.

Complete the following sentences:

1. Specialized functions of the pacing and conduction system include _____ impulse formation and variable _____ velocity.

2. Relatively rapid automatic pacing in the _____ normally dominates the slower intrinsic pacing activity of the _____ junction and _____ fibers.

3. Conduction velocity is slow in the _____ _____ , but rapid in the _____ _____ network.

Review. Automatic impulse formation and variable conduction velocity are special functions of the pacing and conduction system. Impulse formation in the more rapid SA node dominates slower automatic foci in the AV junction and ventricular Purkinje fibers. The AV node conducts slowly; conduction in the His—Purkinje system below the node is rapid.

In reviewing the basic anatomy and function of the pacing and conduction system, we have used the term *electrical activity* as a synonym for depolarization. *Depolarization,* a fundamental response of excitable cells, occurs when cations from fluid around the cell flow across the cell membrane. The positive charge of these ions overcomes the electrically negative state present within the resting cell. The heart's pacing cells undergo depolarization automatically. Other heart muscle cells depolarize only when stimulated. Depolarization spreads from one cell to another—the process of conduction.

When heart muscle cells depolarize, contraction occurs. The contracted state persists until ion flow across cell membranes restores the negative intracellular potential characteristic of the resting muscle cell. This second form of transmembrane ion flow is *repolarization.* Before repolarization, the depolarized cell is in a *refractory period,* incapable of response to stimulation.

EKG waves are a record of electrical forces developed during depolarization or repolarization of large cell masses—the atria and ventricles. Each wave represents a complex summation of myriad small forces developed by individual cells. Depolarization and repolarization forces from lesser groups of cells, such as the nodes and bundles of the pacing and conduction system, cannot be detected by electrodes on the body surface. A specially designed electrode placed through a vein into the heart chambers is capable of recording small electrical forces that result from depolarization of the His bundle.

Complete the following sentences:

1. During depolarization, the cardiac cell loses the _____ internal electrical charge characteristic of the resting state because an influx of _____ occurs across the cell membrane.

2. The electrical change associated with relaxation of a contracted muscle fiber is _____ .

3. During a normal cardiac cycle, the _____ process spreads through the _____ node to the _____ and its branches.

4. _____ must occur before a contracted muscle fiber can again respond to stimulation.

Review. Cation influx during depolarization eliminates the negative intracellular change present in resting cells. Repolarization corresponds to muscle fiber relaxation and must occur before a contracted fiber can respond to a new stimulus. Depolarization in the conduction system spreads through the AV node to the His bundle and its branches.

Table 1–1 Events of the Cardiac Cycle

Electrical Event	Hemodynamic Event
SA node depolarizes	—
Atrial muscle depolarizes	Atria contract
Conduction is delayed in AV node	Ventricles fill
Depolarization spreads through His bundle and its branches	—
Ventricular muscle depolarizes	Ventricles contract
Ventricles repolarize	Ventricles relax and fill

ELECTRICAL AND HEMODYNAMIC EVENTS OF THE CARDIAC CYCLE

Study Table 1-1 closely. This table lists the sequence of electrical events during a single heartbeat and the corresponding hemodynamic events. These events are governed by the pacing and conduction system.

The events of Table 1-1 are represented in the EKG by characteristic waves and intervals, illustrated in Figure 1-2. The *P wave* records electrical forces of atrial depolarization. An atrial repolarization wave is not ordinarily visible because it is small and hidden by the QRS complex. During the *PR interval* (PRI), depolarization spreads through the atria, the AV node, the His bundle, and the bundle branches. The *QRS complex* records ventricular depolarization forces. The ventricles remain depolarized during the *ST segment*. The *T wave* records electrical forces of ventricular repolarization. In Lessons 5 through 8, you will learn about each wave and interval in detail.

Remember that EKG waves give no direct information about the effectiveness of cardiac contraction. In advanced heart disease, the EKG may record a normal sequence of electrical events at a time when

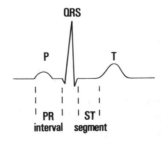

Figure 1-2

the heart is not pumping. This condition, called *electromechanical dissociation,* is a form of cardiac arrest.

Complete the following sentences:

1. The PRI begins at the onset of _____ contraction and ends at the onset of ventricular _____ .

2. T waves occur as the ventricles _____ and _____ .

3. During the ST segment, the _____ have contracted and are _____ to new stimuli.

4. A patient has a deathlike appearance and no detectable pulse, but the cardiac monitor continues to show regular EKG complexes. This condition is _____ _____ .

Review. The PRI begins at the onset of atrial contraction and ends at the onset of ventricular contraction. The T wave corresponds to ventricular depolarization and relaxation. Sustained ventricular contraction during the ST segment leaves the depolarized ventricles refractory to new stimuli. The patient described in sentence 4 illustrates electromechanical dissociation.

Electrical events during a series of cardiac cycles may be conveniently illustrated using a "ladder diagram," each horizontal space on the ladder corresponding to a heart structure. Examine Figure 1-3, a two-space ladder with vertical lines that represent four regular depolarizations of the SA node (SAN), each followed by conduction of depolarization through the atria (A). In Figure 1-4, the diagram illustrates

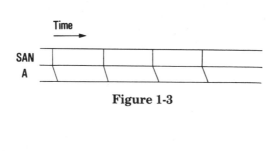

Figure 1-3

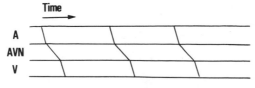

Figure 1-4

three cardiac cycles. Slow conduction through the AV node (AVN) is represented by a sloping line. The ventricles (V) depolarize rapidly.

1. In Figure 1-5, the ladder diagram indicates that _____ of the SA node is irregular. The horizontal space representing the _____ is not labeled.

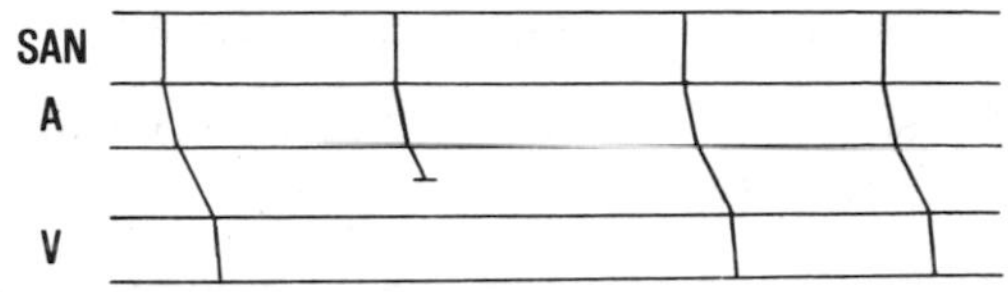

Figure 1-5

2. During the second cycle, the _____ do not depolarize.

Review. Figure 1-5 illustrates irregular depolarization of the SA node. The unlabeled third horizontal space represents the AV node. Ventricular depolarization does not occur during the second cycle on the diagram.

Lesson 2

Limb Leads / Lead Axes in the Frontal Plane

In the early years of the 20th century, Professor Willem Einthoven began for the first time to record human electrocardiograms systematically. He used three leads, now standard limb leads I, II, and III, recorded from electrodes placed on the right arm (RA), left arm (LA), and left leg (LL). These leads are bipolar. For each pair of electrodes, one is designated positive and the other negative, as follows:

Lead I: RA−   LA +
Lead II: RA−   LL +
Lead III: LA−   LL +

Historically, the electrical polarity and interrelationships of the bipolar limb leads have been illustrated by the Einthoven triangle, as diagramed in Figure 2-1.

During the cardiac cycle, a series of electrical forces from the heart results in a changing electrical field present throughout the body. These forces are not uniformly distributed to the body surface. In Figure 2-1, the arrow represents an instantaneous force directed principally toward the LA electrode position. Each cardiac electrical force

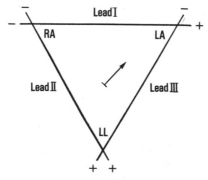

Figure 2-1   Einthoven triangle.

thus causes a transient difference in electrical potentials sensed at each limb electrode. EKG waves are an amplified continuous record of these potential differences as they develop, moment by moment, during the heart cycle.

Examine the position of lead I in the Einthoven triangle. This lead records differences in electrical potentials that are sensed at the RA and LA electrodes. The lead I axis, or spatial orientation, is horizontal.

The principle that governs the relation between the direction of an electrical force and its recorded appearance in lead I is a fundamental aspect of electrocardiography. Figure 2-2 illustrates this principle. Arrows A, B, and C represent hypothetical electrical forces, indicating the size and direction of the force at a moment in time. The record of each instantaneous force on lead I will show its size and direction. Force A, directed toward the positive pole of lead I (LA), will be recorded as an upright, or positive, deflection, with a height of six units. Study the height and direction of the lead I deflection for instantaneous forces B and C. Force C is recorded as a downward, or negative, deflection.

Clearly, the widely varied instantaneous cardiac electrical forces will not ordinarily have a direction exactly parallel to lead I, but an arrow showing the direction of a force will indicate its rightward or leftward displacement from the zero point of the lead I axis. This displacement determines the size and direction of the lead I deflection.

In Figure 2-3, examine arrow A, which represents an instantaneous force directed downward and to the left. Lead I will record only the extent to which force A points to the left. This component of force A is directed toward the positive pole of lead I and it is four units in magnitude. Arrow B represents an instantaneous force that is perpendicular to lead I. Because force B is not displaced to the right or left of the lead I zero point, it will cause no lead I deflection. Correspondingly,

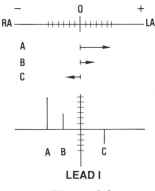

Figure 2-2

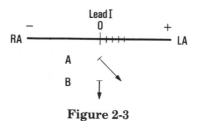

Figure 2-3

a 12-lead EKG may show an electrical force or wave in some leads, but not in other leads to which the force is perpendicular.

Complete the following sentences:

1. For EKG lead I, the _____ _____ electrode is arbitrarily considered positive.

2. An electrical force directed toward the RA will cause a _____ deflection in lead I.

3. Electrical force A in Figure 2-4 will be recorded in lead I by a deflection that is _____ in direction and _____ units in magnitude. The lead I deflection representing force B will be _____ in direction and _____ units in magnitude.

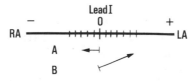

Figure 2-4

Review. The LA electrode is positive for lead I, and a force toward the RA will cause a downward, or negative, lead I deflection. Force A in Figure 2-4 is parallel to the lead I axis and will cause a negative deflection of three units. Force B is displaced six units to the left of the zero point for the lead I axis and will cause a positive deflection.

Interrelationships of the standard limb leads can be conveniently illustrated by arrangement of the lead axes as shown in Figure 2-5, the triaxial reference diagram. The intersection of the lead axes corresponds to the zero point, or baseline, for each lead. The position of each lead's axis is indicated by the angle it forms with the lead I axis, with positive angles measured clockwise.

The lead axes for leads I, II, and III lie in a single plane that corresponds anatomically to the frontal plane. Electrical forces in the

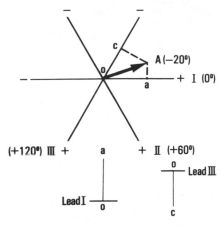

Figure 2-5 Triaxial reference diagram.

frontal plane may be directed rightward, leftward, upward, or downward. In Figure 2-5, arrow A represents an instantaneous force directed upward and to the right in the frontal plane. We can describe the direction, or axis, of force A by measuring the angle it forms with lead I. This angle of 20° is given a negative sign because it is measured above the lead I axis.

Force A in Figure 2-5 is displaced by distance oa from the zero point of lead I and toward the positive pole for this lead. It is displaced by distance oc toward the negative pole of lead III. These displacements determine the magnitude and direction of the deflection, representing force A in leads I and III.

Complete the following sentences:

1. The axis of lead II is _____°.

2. An instantaneous electrical force that is upward and precisely vertical has an axis of _____° in the frontal plane and will cause no deflection on lead _____.

3. An instantaneous force directed toward the negative pole of lead _____ will have an axis of −60°.

Review. The lead II axis is +60°, measured clockwise from the lead I axis. A vertical upward force has an axis of −90° and will not be represented on lead I because it is not displaced from the zero point for this lead. A force directed toward the negative pole of lead III has an axis of −60°.

Additional limb leads aVR, aVL, and aVF are also used to display cardiac electrical forces in the frontal plane. These leads, introduced by

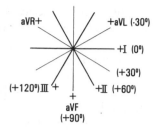

Figure 2-6   Hexaxial reference diagram.

Dr. Emmanuel Goldberger in 1942, are unipolar (V). Each lead records the electrical potential difference between a single limb electrode and an electronically derived zero potential. The unipolar limb leads are also augmented (a); that is, the waves they record are magnified by nearly 50% so that their amplitude is comparable to wave amplitudes displayed in the bipolar limb leads. The designation aVR indicates an augmented unipolar lead recorded from the RA.

Axes for unipolar limb leads may be superimposed on the bipolar lead axes to form the hexaxial reference diagram illustrated in Figure 2-6. The axis for each unipolar lead is represented by a line drawn from its positive pole position through the zero point of the diagram. Note that, with the exception of aVR, positive poles for the limb leads are adjacent. Electrical forces directed downward and to the left will tend to cause a positive, or upright, deflection in these leads, but a negative deflection in aVR.

In Figure 2-6, observe that each unipolar limb lead axis is perpendicular to a bipolar lead axis. Lead aVF and lead I, for example, have mutually perpendicular axes. Examine Figure 2-7, which illustrates that the lead I axis forms a boundary between the positive and negative zones for lead aVF in the frontal plane. All electrical forces directed below the lead I axis will be positive for aVF. Similarly, aVL divides the

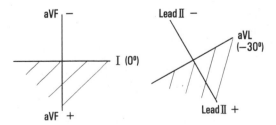

Figure 2-7

frontal plane into positive and negative zones for lead II. All electrical forces directed above −30° will be represented in lead II as a negative deflection.

Complete the following sentences:

1. In Figure 2-8, the _____ , or spatial direction, of electrical force A is nearly parallel to lead _____ and, therefore, approximately _____ °. Of the three lead axes shown, force A will be represented by an upward deflection in leads _____ and _____ .

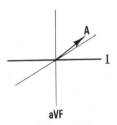

Figure 2-8

2. Lead aVR forms a boundary between positive and negative zones for lead _____ in the frontal plane.

3. An electrical force that causes a positive deflection in both aVF and lead I will lie between _____ ° and _____ °.

Review. Force A in Figure 2-8 has an axis of approximately −30° because it is nearly parallel to lead aVL. This force will be positive in leads I and aVL. Positive and negative zones for lead III are bounded by the aVR axis. The zone of the frontal plane that is positive for both aVF and lead I lies between 0° and +90°.

Lesson 3

Chest Leads / Cardiac Electrical Forces in the Horizontal Plane

In Lesson 2, you learned principles that govern the limb lead display of electrical forces that lie approximately in the frontal plane. Electrical forces from the heart are not confined to a single plane, but have direction and magnitude in three dimensions of space. The six precordial chest leads V_1 through V_6 display components of cardiac forces that lie approximately in the horizontal, or transverse, plane.

Routine chest leads, introduced by Dr. F. N. Wilson in 1944, are unipolar (V). Like the unipolar limb leads, each chest lead is positive at its electrode position with respect to a zero reference level. Recording electrodes are placed in the fourth intercostal space to the right (V_1) and left (V_2) of the sternal border. V_4 electrode position is in the fifth intercostal space at the left midclavicular line. V_3 electrode lies between V_2 and V_4. V_5 and V_6 are lateral to V_4 in the left anterior axillary line and the left midaxillary line, respectively. Additional chest leads are sometimes helpful; in children, a lead V_3R is commonly recorded from an electrode position comparable in V_3, but to the right of the sternum. Unlike the limb leads, chest lead electrodes are commonly positioned incorrectly, either inadvertently or unavoidably in patients with excess adipose tissue, large breasts, bandages, or other chest wall abnormality. Interpretation of the chest leads must always take into account the possibility of a lead placement error.

Examine Figure 3-1, a cross-sectional diagram of the thorax showing approximate electrode positions for leads V_1 through V_6 as viewed from above. Lead axes for the chest leads may be constructed by connecting each electrode position, or positive pole, with a zero point at midthorax. For the chest leads, Figure 3-1 is generally comparable to the hexaxial reference diagram of the limb lead axes, but considerably less accurate. Note that the V_2 axis is approximately perpendicular to the lead V_6 axis.

The unipolar chest leads record electrical force components that

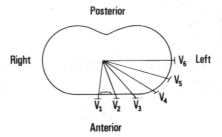

Figure 3-1 Chest lead axes.

are directed anteriorly, posteriorly, rightward, or leftward. In Figure 3-2, examine the diagram of instantaneous force A and its relation to lead axes V_2 and V_6. Force A is directed anteriorly and slightly to the left. Its anterior displacement toward the positive pole of V_2 is large. Its leftward displacement toward the positive pole of V_6 is small. Force B, directed principally to the left and slightly posteriorly, will be represented by a large positive wave in V_6 and a negative wave in V_2.

Complete the following sentences:

1. An electrical force that causes a _____ deflection in lead V_1 will be directed away from the anterior chest wall.

2. An electrical force that causes a positive deflection in leads V_2 and V_6 will cause a _____ deflection in lead V_3.

3. If an electrical force causes a negative deflection in both V_2 and V_6, its direction is _____ and _____ in the horizontal plane.

Review. Electrical forces directed away from the anterior chest wall will cause negative deflections in V_1. If a force is positive with respect to V_2 and V_6, it must also be positive in V_3, V_4, and V_5. A posterior and rightward force will cause negative deflections in both V_2 and V_6.

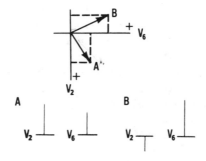

Figure 3-2

Lesson 4

Relation of EKG Leads to Left Ventricular Anatomy

Cardiac disease in adults affects principally the left ventricle (LV). Hypertension, coronary artery disease (CAD), and aortic valve disease are common causes of LV hypertrophy or injury that may lead to major abnormalities of the QRS complex, the ST segment, and the T wave. In patients with CAD, localized ventricular injury occurs, and its location in the ventricular wall determines which EKG leads will display the resulting abnormality of cardiac electrical forces. The relationships between LV anatomy and EKG lead position are not precise, but the concept of this relationship is used regularly in EKG interpretation.

Examine Figure 4-1, a diagrammatic anterior view of the LV, which has a roughly conical shape, with its apex oriented to the left and slightly downward. The anteriorly positioned, thin-walled right ventricle (RV) is not illustrated. The interventricular septum forms most of the anterior LV wall.

Outlined in Figure 4-1 are four major anatomic zones of the LV:

1. Anteroseptal or anterior.
2. Posterior.
3. Anterolateral.
4. Inferior.

Except for the posterior wall, each LV zone corresponds to a group of EKG leads that display the principal EKG abnormalities resulting from injury to that zone.

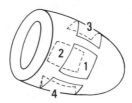

Figure 4-1   Anatomic zones of left ventricle.

Figure 4-2 illustrates an anatomic grouping of EKG leads in the frontal and horizontal planes. The inferior zone, corresponding to leads II, III, and aVF, and the anteroseptal zone, corresponding to leads V_1 and V_2, are well represented in routine leads. The posterior LV wall is not directly represented because routine lead electrodes are not positioned on the posterior thorax. Some LV zones, such as the posterolateral wall, tend to be "silent" because the EKG may remain normal when LV injury is localized to these zones.

Complete the following sentences:

1. As viewed in the frontal plane, the anterolateral LV zone is approximately opposite to the _____ zone.

2. Anteroseptal LV injury causes EKG changes that are principally evident in the _____ plane leads _____ and

   _____ .

3. The limb leads that directly reflect _____ wall injury are II and III and _____ .

4. EKG abnormalities due to _____ zone LV injury tend to be evident in both frontal and horizontal plane leads.

Review.   The anterolateral and inferior zones are approximately opposite in the frontal plane. Leads V_1 and V_2 reflect horizontal plane EKG abnormalities due to anteroseptal LV injury. Leads II, III, and aVF reflect inferior wall injury. Anterolateral injury tends to cause abnormalities in frontal plane leads a VL and I and in horizontal plane leads V_5 and V_6.

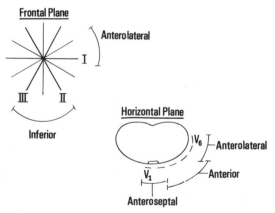

Figure 4-2   Anatomic groups of EKG leads.

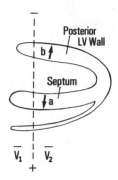

Figure 4-3

The posterior LV zone has an important relation to anteroseptal leads V_1 and V_2. Examine Figure 4-3, a diagram of the LV wall as seen in horizontal cross-section viewed from above. The diagram includes an electrical axis positioned with its positive pole between leads V_1 and V_2. Note that electrical events in the posterior wall are anatomically related to the negative pole of this axis. For this reason, leads V_1 and V_2 may display abnormal waves due to posterior wall LV injury.

Recall that the Purkinje network of the ventricular conduction system lies in the subendocardial region of the LV wall. Ventricular depolarization, therefore, begins in the endocardial layers and spreads to the epicardium, as indicated by arrows a and b on Figure 4-3. These arrows are opposite in direction. When oppositely directed forces develop simultaneously, they tend to cancel each other. Because of such cancellation of opposing forces, the QRS complex theoretically records about 25% of the total electrical forces developed during LV depolarization.

Another issue concerns the display of an electrical force in EKG lead groups that are anatomically opposite to each other. The arrow in Figure 4-4 illustrates an electrical force directed toward the positive

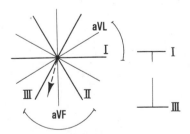

Figure 4-4

poles of inferior leads, but toward the negative poles of anterolateral leads. When inferior wall injury causes an abnormal deflection in II, III, and aVF, a corresponding oppositely directed deflection often appears in I and aVL. These are termed *reciprocal changes*. The inferior lead deflection and the anterolateral lead deflection are reciprocal, or mutual, records of the same electrical force.

Complete the following sentences:

1. A horizontal plane electrical force directed posteriorly will be represented by a _____ deflection in V_1 and V_2.

2. A frontal plane electrical force directed toward $+120°$ will be parallel to the lead _____ axis and will be represented by a _____ deflection in lead aVL.

Review. A posteriorly directed horizontal plane electrical force will be oriented toward the negative pole of the axes for leads V_1 and V_2 and will be represented by a negative reflection in these leads. A force directed toward $+120°$ will be parallel to lead III and will be represented by a negative reciprocal deflection in lead aVL.

Lesson 5

Normal P Waves / Use of EKG Graph Paper to Measure Wave Dimensions and Rate

P waves display electrical forces that develop during atrial depolarization. In the frontal plane, atrial forces are normally directed downward and to the left toward the positive pole of all the limb leads except aVR. Normal P waves are usually upright in these leads. Their configuration in the limb leads is smoothly rounded or slightly notched, as illustrated in Figure 5-1. Identification of P waves is ordinarily a first step in routine EKG interpretation.

P wave dimensions can be conveniently measured on EKG graph paper using lead I, II, or III. Choose the lead that has the clearest wave form, usually lead II. The height of a P wave, or other upright wave, is measured from the top of the EKG baseline to the top of the wave. An EKG record is ordinarily calibrated, or "standardized," so that a 10-mm vertical deflection is equivalent to an amplifier output of 1 mV. In Figure 5-2, the P wave height, c, is slightly more than 1 mm, corresponding to 0.1 mV. At standard calibration, P wave height normally should not exceed 2.5 to 3.0 mm.

P wave duration indicates the time interval required for depolarization to spread from the SA node throughout both atria. The duration of a positive wave is measured at the top of the baseline, from point a to

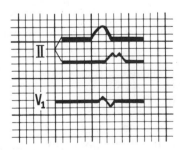

Figure 5-1   Normal P wave configuration.

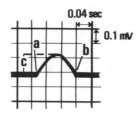

Figure 5-2 Measurement of P wave dimensions.

point b in Figure 5-2. At usual recording paper speed of 25 mm/sec, the width of each small square measures 0.04 sec. The duration of the P wave in Figure 5-2 is 2.5 small squares, or 0.10 sec. Normal P wave duration is 0.11 sec or less. A P wave that is three small squares or more in width is abnormal.

In the horizontal plane leads, only the P wave in V_1 is routinely examined. In this lead, the P wave usually shows a small positive initial component followed by a small negative component, a biphasic contour illustrated in Figure 5-1. Remember that depolarization begins in the right atrium, the location of the SA node, and spreads to the left atrium. The initial upward P wave component in V_1 corresponds to right atrial depolarization and the terminal downward component corresponds to left atrial depolarization. The left atrial component should not exceed 1 mm in depth or 1 mm (0.04 sec) in duration.

Complete the following sentences:

1. Normal P wave duration, usually best measured in
   lead _____ , should not exceed _____ sec, or slightly
   less than _____ small squares on EKG paper at standard
   recording speed of _____ mm/sec.

2. P wave amplitude should normally be less
   than _____ to _____ mm as measured in
   the _____ lead group when standard calibration is used,
   with the height of _____ small squares equal to 1 mV.

3. Normally, P wave forces are directed downward
   and _____ , toward the _____ pole of lead II and
   the _____ pole of lead aVR.

4. In lead V_1, the normal P wave has a _____ shape with a
   negative component that corresponds to _____ atrial
   depolarization.

Review. P wave duration should not exceed 0.11 sec, slightly less than three small squares at a paper speed of 25 mm/sec. P wave amplitude in the inferior leads should be less than 2.5 to 3.0 mm, when 10 mm equals 1 mV. Normal P waves have a leftward and downward orientation, toward the positive pole of lead II and the negative pole of aVR. In lead V_1 the normal P wave is commonly biphasic, with a terminal negative component of left atrial depolarization.

During normal heart rhythm, P waves reflect the rate of spontaneous impulse formation in the SA node. In adult patients at rest, the heart rate during normal sinus rhythm is between 50 or 60 beats per minute (bpm) and 100 bpm. Normal sinus rhythm in adults is nearly regular; the P-to-P interval between consecutive P waves varies by less than 10%. P wave rates below 50 or 60 bpm indicate sinus bradycardia (SB), and rates above 100 bpm indicate sinus tachycardia (ST). Excessive variation in the P-to-P interval indicates sinus arrhythmia.

Several features of EKG graph paper are helpful in measuring heart rate. In Figure 5-3, note the small vertical lines at the paper's upper border. At standard paper speed of 25 mm/sec, these lines measure a 3-sec interval. The heavy vertical lines of the graph measure 0.2 sec, or five times 0.04 sec.

Figure 5-3 shows a series of P waves. Use EKG calipers to determine that the P-to-P intervals are regular. Measure these intervals from the onset of each P wave to the onset of the next wave. What is the duration of this P-to-P interval in seconds? When P waves are regular at an interval of five large squares, or 1 sec, their rate is 60 bpm. Learn the following intervals and the corresponding rates for regular heart rhythms:

Six large squares (1.2 sec)	50 bpm
Four large squares (0.8 sec)	75 bpm
Three large squares (0.6 sec)	100 bpm
Two large squares (0.4 sec)	150 bpm

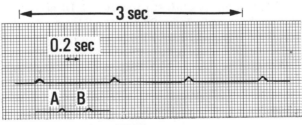

Figure 5-3

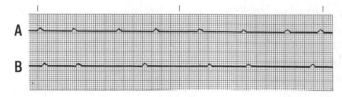

Figure 5-4

When heart rhythm is regular, the rate per minute may be calculated by dividing the number of small squares in the P-to-P interval into 1500, the number of small squares per minute at a paper speed of 25 mm/sec. In Figure 5-3, the P-to-P interval is 25 small squares and the rate is 1500 divided by 25, or 60 bpm.

When heart rhythm is irregular, the rate per minute may be estimated by a 6-sec wave count, using two 3-sec intervals as measured by the vertical lines on the paper's upper border. In Figure 5-4, for each series of irregular P waves, select a wave under or near the first small vertical line. Beginning with the next wave, count the number of waves in a 6-sec interval and multiply this number by 10 to estimate the rate in bpm. For series A, the rate is approximately 70 bpm.

Complete the following sentences:

1. In Figure 5-3, the interval from wave A to B is
   _____ small squares, or _____ sec, corresponding to
   a rate of _____ bpm.

2. When SA node depolarization occurs every _____ second,
   the resulting P-to-P interval is 14 small squares and the
   corresponding heart rate is _____ bpm.

3. For series B of Figure 5-4, the estimated P wave rate
   is _____ bpm, and the rhythm is irregular, indicating both
   sinus _____ and sinus _____.

Review. Waves A and B on Figure 5-3 are separated by nine small squares, equivalent to 0.36 sec at a paper speed of 25 mm/sec and a heart rate of 166 bpm. A P-to-P interval of 14 squares, or 0.56 sec, corresponds to a rate of 107 bpm. Series B of Figure 5-4 illustrates both sinus bradycardia and sinus arrhythmia at an irregular rate of 50 bpm.

Lesson 6

Normal QRS Complexes / The QRS Axis

Normal QRS complexes reflect the pattern of *ventricular depolarization* as electrical impulses, conducted rapidly through the His bundle branches and the subendocardial Purkinje network, activate ventricular muscle. Depolarization spreads from the base of the ventricle toward its apex. Correspondingly, the main QRS force is normally directed downward and to the left in the frontal plane. Depolarization of the ventricular muscle mass normally requires 0.10 sec or less, the normal QRS complex duration.

Examine Figure 6-1, a cross-sectional diagram of the LV as seen from above, showing hypothetical depolarization forces. Arrow A represents an initial septal force that develops as depolarization spreads from the left bundle branch across the ventricular septum, directed anteriorly and to the right. Arrow B represents the main depolarization force from the LV wall, which has a posterior and leftward direction. This force develops 0.01 to 0.02 sec after the initial septal force. Right ventricular forces are relatively small and cannot be identified in the normal QRS complex.

Figure 6-1 illustrates the display of QRS forces A and B in leads V_1 and V_6. The initial anterior and rightward septal force corresponds to a small positive deflection in V_1 and small negative deflection in V_6. Force B, directed posteriorly and to the left toward the positive pole of

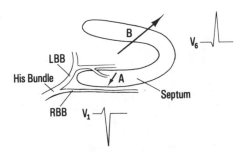

Figure 6-1 Hypothetical LV depolarization forces in the horizontal plane.

V_6 and away from the positive pole of V_1, then dominates the QRS complex.

Examine Figure 6-2, which illustrates the terms used to describe the configuration of QRS complexes. The letters used to designate individual waves are

Q—negative deflection before an R wave
R—first positive deflection
S—negative deflection after an R wave
QS—negative deflection in absence of an R wave
R′—second positive deflection after an S wave

In older adults, R or S wave amplitude should normally not exceed 20 mm (2.0 mV) in the limb leads. S waves in V_{1-2} and R waves in V_{5-6} should not exceed 30 mm (3.0 mV). Total QRS amplitude (R wave plus S wave) should be at least 5.0 mm (0.5 mV) in at least one of the limb leads.

Complete the following sentences:

1. An abnormal QRS complex may indicate dysfunction of the _____ _____ system or an abnormality of _____ muscle.

2. During normal LV depolarization, the main QRS force is oriented _____ and _____ in the frontal plane.

3. The initial QRS force originates in the ventricular _____ and is represented by a small _____ deflection in lead V_1.

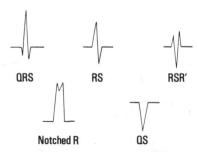

QRS   RS   RSR′

Notched R   QS

Figure 6-2   Nomenclature for QRS wave forms.

4. Normal QRS duration is _____ second or less. Except
   in young patients, R or S wave amplitude should not
   exceed _____ mm in the limb leads or _____ mm in
   the chest leads.

Review. QRS abnormalities may result from dysfunction of the His-
Purkinje system or from a ventricular muscle abnormality. LV depolarization spreads from base to apex, and the main QRS forces are correspondingly directed downward and leftward. A small positive deflection
in V_1 represents an initial QRS force from the ventricular septum. QRS
duration is normally 0.10 sec or less. R or S wave amplitude should not
exceed 20 mm in the limb leads or 30 mm in the chest leads at standard
calibration (10 mm = 1.0 mV).

Figure 6-3 shows the normal appearance of QRS complexes in the
horizontal plane, indicating electrode positions for the chest leads as
viewed from above. Note that R wave amplitude steadily increases from
right to left across the precordium. This important feature is termed *R
wave progression.* Correspondingly, S wave amplitude gradually diminishes. At some point on the precordium, called the *transition zone,* R and
S wave amplitudes are approximately equal. Normally, the transition
zone lies between leads V_2 and V_5.

Examine series A of Figure 6-4, in which V_5 is the transition
complex. A leftward shift of the transition zone to V_5 or V_6 is termed
clockwise rotation, as suggested by the clock diagram. Conversely, a
rightward shift of the transition zone to V_1 or V_2, as in series B of Figure

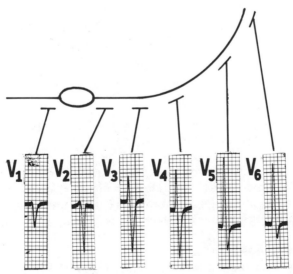

Figure 6-3   Normal QRS complexes in chest leads.

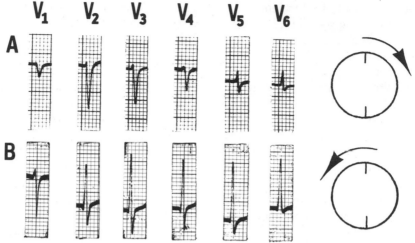

Figure 6-4 QRS complexes showing (A) clockwise and (B) counterclockwise rotation.

6-4, is termed *counterclockwise rotation*. Note that in series A the R wave amplitude is low in V_2, V_3, and V_4. When R wave amplitude does not increase as expected in the sequence of precordial leads, the pattern is termed *delayed* (or "poor") *R wave progression*. If R wave amplitude decreases, so that R waves in lead V_2 or V_3 are smaller than in V_1, the pattern is called *reversed R wave progression*.

Complete the following sentences:

1. In lead V_5 of series A, Figure 6-4, the QRS complex is
   _____ because the _____ and _____ have
   equal amplitude.

2. Small R waves in leads V_2 and V_3, only slightly taller than the
   V_1 R wave, form the pattern called _____ progression.

3. If the R and S waves in lead V_2 have the same amplitude,
   _____ rotation is present.

Review. The R and S waves are equal in transitional QRS complex V_5 of series A. When R wave amplitude does not increase as expected from lead V_1 to lead V_3 or V_4, delayed (or poor) R wave progression is present. A transitional QRS complex in lead V_2 is typical of counterclockwise rotation.

Figure 6-5 illustrates the relationship between QRS forces in the frontal plane and their display in leads I and aVF. In this example, initial force A, directed upward and to the right, is represented by a Q

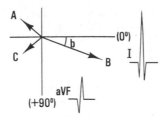

Figure 6-5   Hypothetical LV depolarization forces in the frontal plane.

wave in both leads. Normal Q waves do not exceed 0.02 sec in duration, or 0.03 sec in lead III. Among normal subjects, the direction of initial QRS forces varies considerably and individual limb leads often do not display a Q wave. Force B of Figure 6-5, the main QRS force, is directed downward and to the left in this illustration, a common normal orientation that results in R waves in both leads I and aVF. Because force B is directed principally toward the positive pole of lead I, R wave height is maximal in this lead. Angle b, between force B and the lead I axis, is approximately 20° and measures the orientation, or axis, of force B in the frontal plane. The *frontal plane axis of a QRS complex* is determined by the direction of its largest positive force and will be close to the axis of the limb lead displaying the tallest R wave.

Figure 6-6 illustrates the principal frontal plane QRS forces for two subjects X and Y. The QRS force for patient X forms almost a right angle with the lead I axis. This subject's QRS axis is +85°. For subject Y, the main QRS force forms an angle of 45° above the lead I axis. This subject has a QRS axis of −45°.

Complete the following sentences:

1. The main force of a QRS complex is exactly vertical and downward. This complex has a mean QRS axis of _____ ° and will show a large _____ wave in lead _____ .

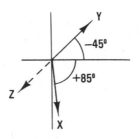

Figure 6-6

2. When the frontal plane leads show a large R wave only in lead II, the mean QRS axis is approximately ＿＿＿＿＿＿°.

3. The QRS axis for subject Z in Figure 6-6 is ＿＿＿＿＿＿°.

Review. A vertical and downward QRS complex has an axis of +90° and lead aVF will display a large R wave. A QRS axis oriented toward lead II is +60°. Subject Z has a QRS axis of +135°, opposite to the −45° axis of subject Y.

Estimation of frontal plane QRS axis based on the hexaxial reference diagram is a routine step in EKG interpretation. Figure 6-7 illustrates the normal range for QRS axis in adults, −30° to +105° and indicates the terms used to describe abnormal QRS axis directions. *Left axis deviation* (LAD), above −30°, is a common finding that may result from fibrosis of the His—Purkinje system involving predominately the anterior fascicle of the left bundle branch (LAFB). In older subjects, this abnormality is often innocuous. *Right axis deviation* (RAD) is uncommon.

To detect LAD with QRS axis of −30° or above, examine the lead II QRS complex. Recall that lead aVL, with −30° axis, forms a boundary between negative and positive zones for lead II. Figure 6-8 illustrates this relationship. If the QRS complex is positive in lead II, LAD is not present. The R and S waves in lead II are equal (equiphasic complex) when the QRS axis is −30°. Occasionally, an EKG may show an equiphasic complex in every limb lead, requiring a diagnosis of indeterminate QRS axis.

Complete the following sentences:

1. An EKG shows left axis deviation when the QRS complex is positive in lead I and ＿＿＿＿＿＿ in lead II.

2. When the QRS complex is equiphasic in lead II and positive in lead I, the QRS axis is directed toward the positive pole of lead ＿＿＿＿＿＿ at ＿＿＿＿＿＿°.

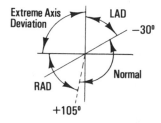

Figure 6-7 Normal and abnormal QRS axis positions in the frontal plane.

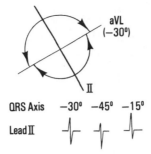

Figure 6-8 Relationship of lead II QRS complex to LAD.

3. When lead I shows an equiphasic QRS complex, the QRS axis is perpendicular to lead I and may be _____ ° or _____ °.

4. When lead III shows the tallest R wave in the limb leads, QRS axis is approximately _____ ° and _____ axis deviation is present.

Review. When the QRS complex is positive in lead I and negative in lead II, its axis lies between −30° and −90°, and LAD is present. An equiphasic QRS in lead II is consistent with QRS axis of either −30° or +150°; a positive QRS in lead I confirms an axis of −30°, toward the positive pole of aVL. When the lead I QRS is equiphasic, the QRS axis may be +90° or −90°. When the lead III R wave is tallest, RAD of +120° is present.

Lesson 7

Normal PR Interval/ Functions of the AV Node

In Lessons 5 and 6, you learned the characteristics of normal P waves and QRS complexes, methods for estimating heart rate from the EKG, and a method for estimating frontal plane QRS axis. Another routine measurement in EKG interpretation is the *PRI*, the time interval from the onset of atrial depolarization to the onset of ventricular depolarization. PRI duration depends principally on the function of the AV node, where slow conduction normally delays transmission of atrial electrical activity on its path to the His bundle and the ventricles.

Examine Figure 7-1. The PRI is measured from point a, the P wave onset, to point b, the onset of the QRS complex. Note that the PRI ends at onset of the Q wave when one is present. Normal duration of the PRI is 0.12 to 0.20 sec. The PRI has two components, the P wave and the PR segment, which is measured from point c to b in Figure 7-1. The usual cause of a prolonged PRI is excessive conduction delay in the AV node. A short PRI suggests enhanced AV conduction, or pre-excitation of the ventricle, possibly through an abnormal rapid conduction pathway that bypasses the AV node.

In Lesson 1, you learned that electrical activity is conducted through both the AV node and the His—Purkinje system before the onset of ventricular depolarization. Using an intracardiac electrode, it is possible to record an electrical potential due to activation of the His

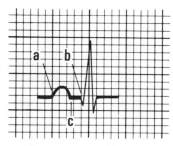

Figure 7-1   PR interval.

bundle. The His bundle potential, or H spike, separates the time interval required for AV node conduction from the time required for His—Purkinje system conduction.

Examine Figure 7-2, which illustrates the relationship between EKG lead II and a simultaneous recording of the His bundle potential, H. The AH interval measures conduction time from the lower right atrium through the AV node. It is more than twice the HV interval, which measures conduction time beyond the His bundle. Abnormal conduction delays may occur in either segment of the AV pathway, but distal conduction delay beyond the His bundle is seldom sufficient to prolong the PRI.

Complete the following sentences:

1. A PRI greater than _____ sec indicates an excessive conduction delay in the _____ _____ .

2. When the interval from onset of the _____ wave to onset of the QRS complex is less than _____ sec, an abnormal conduction pathway bypassing the _____ _____ may be present.

3. Depolarization of the _____ _____ occurs before onset of the P wave, but is not displayed on the EKG.

4. During the PR segment, depolarization occurs in the _____ node and in the _____ system, but is not displayed on the EKG.

Review. Abnormal conduction delay in the AV node is the principal cause of PRI prolongation beyond the normal limit of 0.20 sec. When the PRI is abnormally shortened to less than 0.12 sec, an abnormal conduction pathway bypassing the AV node may exist. SA node depolarization, before onset of the P wave, and depolarization of the AV node and

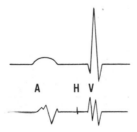

Figure 7-2 His bundle electrogram.

His—Purkinje system, during the PR segment, generate electrical potentials that are too small to be recorded on a routine EKG.

Prolongation of the PRI, termed *first degree AV block,* is a common EKG abnormality that may be an innocuous finding or an indication of important disease. In many patients, the degree of PRI prolongation remains constant and the abnormality is permanent. In other patients, the PRI duration may change from time to time. Usually, the prolongation is slight, but occasionally the PRI may exceed 0.40 sec. The many causes of AV node conduction delay include excessive vagus nerve stimulation and adverse drug effects.

Delayed AV node conduction is readily represented on a ladder diagram. In Figure 7-3, the rate of atrial depolarization is regular. During the series of three cardiac cycles, AV conduction is progressively delayed, indicated by changes in the slope of the line representing AV node depolarization.

When conduction through the AV node and His—Purkinje pathways is normal, every P wave is followed by a QRS complex. The ratio of P waves to QRS complexes, termed the *AV conduction ratio,* is 1:1. If AV conduction is abnormal and every other atrial depolarization fails to penetrate the AV node, the ratio of P waves to QRS complexes is 2:1. The ladder diagram in Figure 7-4 illustrates a 2:1 AV conduction ratio.

When the rate of atrial depolarization is extremely rapid, the AV node has an important role in preventing an equally rapid ventricular rate. For example, often when abnormal atrial depolarization occurs at a rate of 300 bpm, the AV node conducts only every other impulse and the ventricular rate is 150 bpm. The resulting 2:1 AV conduction ratio represents normal function of the AV node.

Complete the following sentences:

1. If only three of every four P waves are followed by a QRS complex, the _____ _____ ratio is _____ to _____ .

2. The _____ nerve may slow both the rate of spontaneous depolarization in the _____ node and the conduction velocity in the _____ node.

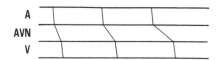

Figure 7-3 Sinus rhythm with onset of delayed AV conduction.

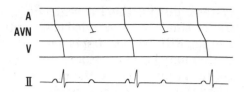

Figure 7-4   Sinus rhythm with 2:1 AV conduction.

Review.   The AV conduction ratio is 4:3 when one of every four P waves is not followed by a QRS complex. The vagus nerve may slow both SA node automaticity and AV node conduction.

Lesson 8

ST Segments, T Waves, and U Waves / The QT Interval

A difficult aspect of EKG interpretation concerns events in the cardiac cycle that follow the QRS complex. In Lesson 1, you learned that T waves measure electrical forces of ventricular repolarization, principally from the LV. They record a complex sum of small electrical forces that originate from individual ventricular muscle cells when ion flow across cell membranes returns them to their resting polarized state. The ST segment precedes the T wave and corresponds to a period of electrical inactivity that immediately follows ventricular depolarization. After the T wave, a small rounded U wave may be recorded; the origin of this wave is not well understood. Figure 8-1 (A) illustrates a normal complex. The J point designates ST segment onset at its junction with the QRS complex. The QT interval (QTI) measures the time between onset of ventricular depolarization and completion of repolarization.

Many forms of heart disease and metabolic disorders may affect T waves and ST segments. T waves show a wide range of normal configuration that overlaps the abnormal spectrum. The normal ST segment is usually flat and on the EKG baseline, but may also be curved and lie slightly above or below the baseline. In contrast to interpretation of P waves and QRS complexes, analysis of ST segments and T waves depends not on measurement of their amplitude and duration, but on assessment of their configuration.

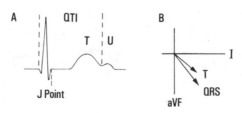

Figure 8-1

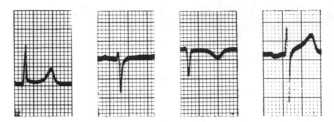

Figure 8-2 Normal ST and T waves configuration.

Figure 8-2 illustrates normal T waves and ST segments. The ST segment may be flat or upsloping. T wave inversion or flattening may be normal in certain EKG leads. Interpretation of T wave inversion commonly depends on the direction of the QRS complex. The T wave direction, or axis, should lie close to the QRS axis, as shown for the frontal plane in Figure 8-1(B). An inverted T wave may be entirely normal in a lead that shows a negative QRS complex.

In Figure 8-3, examine the T waves and their relationship to QRS complexes. The aVR complex normally shows a negative QRS and an inverted T wave. For lead V_1, remember that the QRS complex is normally negative. Normal T waves may be inverted or upright in this lead. In young subjects, inverted T waves may also be present in leads V_2 and V_3, described as the *juvenile T wave pattern*.

Complete the following sentences:

1. In normal older subjects, the T wave direction in lead V_1 may be _____ or _____ , although the QRS complex is regularly _____ in this lead.

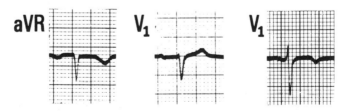

Figure 8-3

2. For each complex in Figure 8-4, describe the ST segment and T wave, indicating whether the T wave is normal or abnormal:

              T Wave   ST Segment

a. _____   _____

b. _____   _____

c. _____   _____

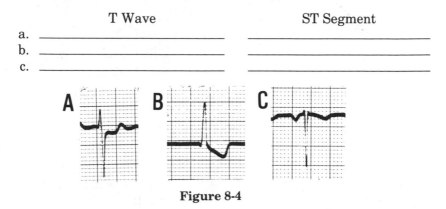

Figure 8-4

3. The complex in Figure 8-4(C) shows a configuration commonly seen in leads _____ and _____ .

Review. T waves in lead V_1 may be upright or inverted in normal older subjects with negative QRS complexes in this lead. Figure 8-4(A) shows a depressed ST segment. The T wave is upright and normal. In Figure 8-4(B), the ST segment is downsloping and depressed; the T wave is abnormally inverted. Figure 8-4(C) shows T inversion in a lead with negative QRS, a normal concordant relationship commonly seen in leads aVR and V_1.

MEASURING THE QTI

The QTI begins at the QRS onset and ends at completion of the T wave. It is closely related to the duration of ventricular systole. Normally, the QTI duration depends on heart rate, for the duration of systole shortens as heart rate increases. Many conditions, especially metabolic disorders and drug effects, tend to prolong this interval.

Examine Figure 8-5(A). The QTI has two principal components, the ST segment and the T wave. Figure 8-5 (B) illustrates a prolonged QTI due to a widened ST segment. In Figure 8-5(C), the QTI is prolonged because the T wave is abnormally wide. In Figure 8-5(D), an abnormally large U wave intersects the T wave, causing apparent prolongation of the QTI, which cannot be measured accurately.

The normal QTI should not exceed 0.40 sec for men or 0.44 sec for women when the heart rate is 60 bpm. A table of normal values, Table 8-1, may be used to determine whether or not the observed QTI is

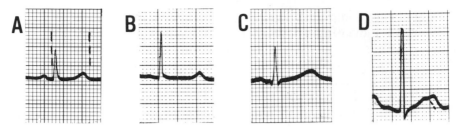

Figure 8-5 Normal and abnormal QTIs.

normal for the observed heart rate. Alternatively, when a regular rhythm is present, the observed QTI may be corrected for heart rate above or below 60 bpm by the following formula:

$$\text{Corrected QTI} = \frac{\text{Observed QTI}}{\text{Square root of R-to-R interval (sec)}}$$

Study the following example:

Observed QTI—0.50 sec $\text{Corrected QTI} = \dfrac{0.50}{\sqrt{1.2}}$

Heart rate—50 bpm

R-to-R interval—1.2 sec $= 0.46 \text{ sec}$

This QTI is abnormally prolonged. The corrected QTI should not exceed the upper limit of normal for a heart rate of 60 bpm.

Complete the following sentences:

1. The QTI is closely related to the duration of ventricular _____ and normally increases in width when heart rate _____ .

2. Each complex of Figure 8-6 was obtained from the EKG of a female subject with a heart rate of 83 bpm. Measure each QTI and state whether the interval is normal or prolonged, referring to Table 8-1.

    a. The QTI of _____ sec is _____ .
    b. The QTI of _____ sec is _____ .
    c. The QTI of _____ sec is _____ .

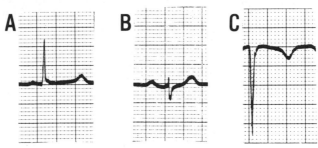

Figure 8-6

3. Each complex of Figure 8-6 except letter _____ suggests a _____ abnormality or drug effect.

Table 8–1   QTI Duration in Men and Women for Varying Heart Rates

| Heart Rate | Upper Limit for Normal QTI (sec) | |
	Men	Women
40	0.49	0.54
50	0.44	0.48
60	0.40	0.44
71	0.37	0.40
83	0.34	0.37
100	0.31	0.34
125	0.28	0.30

Review.   Ventricular systole and the QTI increase in duration as the heart rate slows. In Figure 8-6(A) the QTI is prolonged to 0.50 sec because of a widened ST segment. The prolonged QTI in Figure 8-6(C), is also 0.50 sec. In Figure 8-6(B) the QTI is normal, 0.36 sec, and does not suggest the presence of a metabolic abnormality.

Lesson 9

EKG Artifacts and Recording Errors

An essential preliminary step in EKG interpretation is an evaluation of technical features of the 12-lead tracing. Failure to recognize technical defects or artifacts is potentially a serious source of error. Common technical mistakes include improper electrode placement, erroneous voltage calibration or paper speed setting, and even improper labeling or mounting of the EKG record. *Artifacts* are EKG waves that do not represent electrical activity of the heart. They may appear because of voluntary or involuntary patient movement such as a tremor or hiccough. They may be caused by electrical interference from external sources. An interpreter must be constantly aware of these potential problems.

In Lesson 5, you learned that voltage measurements on EKG paper are calibrated for a 10-mm deflection in response to an amplifier output of 1 mV. A calibration switch permits the EKG technician to adjust this response to 20 mm/mV (double standard) or to 5 mm/mV (half standard). A technically adequate EKG should clearly show its calibration as recorded in a standardization artifact, a square wave corresponding to 1 mV, as shown in Figure 9-1.

Another important technical consideration is paper recording speed. As Figure 9-2 illustrates, a change of paper speed from 25 to 50 mm/sec causes an apparent bradycardia and doubles the width of all EKG waves and intervals, a misleading effect when rapid paper speed has been used inadvertently.

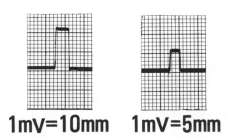

1mV=10mm   1mV=5mm

Figure 9-1   Calibration artifacts.

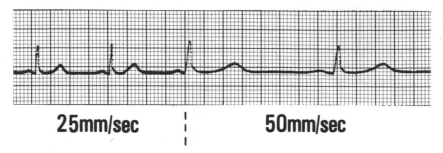

25mm/sec   **50mm/sec**

Figure 9-2 Paper speed effects.

One of the most troublesome technical errors results from incorrect electrode placement. The Einthoven triangle in Figure 9-3 illustrates effects of interchanging RA and LA electrodes. This error causes inversion of lead I (negative and positive poles reversed) and an interchange of leads II and III. P wave inversion in lead I is an important clue to arm lead reversal.

Chest lead connections may also be reversed when these leads are simultaneously recorded. With recording equipment currently in common use, the interchange may involve single chest leads or groups of leads. Chest lead reversal should be suspected when the pattern of R wave progression in leads V_1 to V_6 is bizarre.

Artifacts are usually less subtle than technical errors. When misinterpreted, they are most often mistaken for disorders of heart rhythm. Figure 9-4 illustrates several types of artifact. Because the

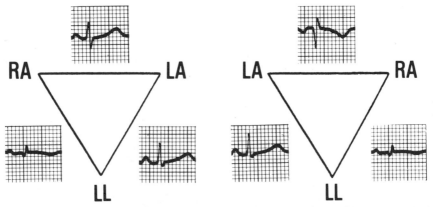

Figure 9-3 Effects of arm lead reversal. Lead I is inverted and leads II and III are interchanged.

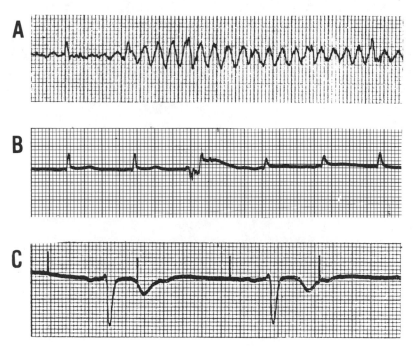

Figure 9-4 EKG artifacts due to (A) tremor, (B) hiccough, and (C) artificial pacemaker.

artifact due to tremor, Figure 9-4(A), was misinterpreted as a rhythm disorder, the patient was inappropriately admitted to an intensive care unit. The pacemaker artifact, Figure 9-4(C), represents the output of an electronic cardiac pacemaker that is malfunctioning.

Complete the following sentences:

1. For a patient with a heart rate of 80 bpm and PRI equal to the upper limit of normal, a paper speed of 50 mm/sec will cause an apparent rate of _____ bpm and the PRI will be _____ sec.

2. When LL and LA electrodes are reversed, the lead recorded as lead I will actually be lead _____ .

3. Arm lead reversal is a common cause of _____ inversion in lead I.

4. When misinterpreted, artifacts are usually mistaken for a disorder of _____ _____ .

Review. For the patient referred to in sentence 1, doubling the paper speed will result in an apparent rate of 40 bpm and PRI of 0.40 sec. LL and LA reversal interchanges leads I and II. P wave inversion in lead I suggests arm lead reversal. Artifacts may be mistaken for heart rhythm disorders.

Outline / Steps in Routine 12-Lead EKG Interpretation

In Lesson 5 through 8, you learned the characteristics of normal EKG waves and intervals. The outline below suggests an organized method for applying this knowledge to identify a normal 12-lead EKG. Normal values are indicated in parentheses. Much of the information needed for this analysis is available in lead II and in two lead groups, V_1–V_2 and V_5–V_6.

1. Preliminary step:
   a. Note patient's age, sex, and clinical diagnosis.
   b. Evaluate technical features of tracing; note voltage calibration artifact (standard calibration 1 mV = 10 mm).
2. Identify P waves in lead II and other limb leads:
   a. Note rhythm regularity.
   b. Determine heart rate (50 or 60 to 100 bpm) using small square count or 6-sec count.
   c. Note P wave width (<0.12 sec) and amplitude (<2.5 to 3.0 mm).
3. Measure PR interval (0.12 to 0.20 sec) and note AV conduction ratio (1 to 1).
4. Analyze QRS complexes:
   a. Determine frontal plane QRS axis ($-30°$ to $+105°$, with upright lead II complex).
   b. Measure maximum QRS width in limb leads (≤0.10 sec).
   c. Measure maximum R or S wave height in limb leads (<20 mm) and in V_1–V_2 (S wave <30 mm) or V_5–V_6 (R wave <30 mm).
   d. Note absence of abnormal Q waves (normal Q wave width ≤0.02 sec, or ≤ 0.03 sec in lead III).
   e. Note R wave progression in chest leads.
5. Analyze ST segments and T waves:
   a. Note ST segments at or near the EKG baseline.
   b. Note upright T waves in leads with positive QRS.
   c. Measure QTI, correcting for heart rate (<0.44 sec for women, <0.40 sec for men at rate 60 bpm).

2 | Abnormal P Waves

Lesson 10

Atrial Automatic Pacing Foci / Retrograde P Waves

In Lesson 5, you learned about normal P wave characteristics, which depend on origin of depolarization in the SA node and its spread through normal atrial conduction pathways. In Lesson 7, you learned that duration of the PRI depends on conduction properties of the AV node as it transmits atrial depolarization to the His bundle in a normal, or antegrade, direction. Lesson 10 considers important abnormalities of P wave timing and configuration that occur when atrial depolarization originates from an automatic pacing focus outside the SA node. Any pacing focus outside the SA node is, by definition, ectopic.

· The normal AV junction contains ectopic pacing cells that depolarize at a regular rate of 40 to 50 bpm. When a junctional focus paces the heart, P wave configuration is often abnormal. During junctional rhythm, atrial depolarization may spread from the AV junction toward the SA node, an opposite, or *retrograde,* direction as compared to normal sinus rhythm. As a result, P waves in leads II and III are inverted. QRS complexes typically have a normal, narrow supraventricular pattern during junctional rhythm. The PRI, which does not depend on slow conduction through the AV node as it does during sinus rhythm, is usually short (<0.12 sec).

During normal sinus rhythm, impulses from the SA node are conducted through the AV junction and suppress the junctional pacemaker. In general, the most rapid supraventricular pacemaker will control, or "capture," the ventricles. If SA node pacing slows excessively, the junctional pacemaker may "escape" SA node dominance and control heart rhythm.

Complete the following sentences:

1. Inverted P waves occur during _____ escape rhythm because of _____ conduction in the atria.

2. Another cause of P wave inversion in lead I is _____ _____ .

3. Normal P wave configuration depends both on origin of

depolarization in the _____ node and normal conduction through _____ tracts.

Review. Junctional escape rhythm may cause P wave inversion due to retrograde atrial conduction. P wave inversion in lead I may result from arm lead reversal. P wave abnormalities may be expected when depolarization originates outside the SA node or when internodal tracts conduct abnormally during sinus rhythm.

When a junctional pacemaker controls the atria by retrograde conduction, three different time relationships are possible between retrograde P waves and QRS complexes. The ladder diagram in Figure 10-1 illustrates that depolarization originates in the AV junction (AVN). In Figure 10-1(A), retrograde conduction to the atria occurs before antegrade conduction to the ventricles. Correspondingly, an inverted retrograde P wave is present before the QRS complex. Note also that the PRI is short. Examine Figure 10-1(B). Note that retrograde conduction and antegrade conduction from the junctional pacing focus occur at the same time. The retrograde P wave is hidden in the QRS complex. Now analyze the P wave and QRS relationship shown in Figure 10-1(C).

Examine Figure 10-1(D). Note that a normal upright P wave follows the QRS complex. In this illustration, the AV junctional pacemaker paces the ventricles, but the sinus node paces the atrium. For this cycle, the atria and the ventricles are activated by separate pacemakers, an example of *AV dissociation.*

Retrograde P waves also may occur when a pacing focus in the ventricle controls heart rhythm. From the ventricular focus, depolarization may spread retrograde through the His-Purkinje system, the AV node, and the atria. Examine Figure 10-2, which shows an electronically paced ventricular rhythm. Each pacing artifact is followed by a QRS complex. A retrograde P wave is present in the ST segment with exception of the fourth complex, during which retrograde conduction to the atria has failed.

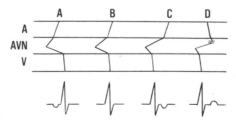

Figure 10-1 Patterns of atrial activation during AV junctional rhythms.

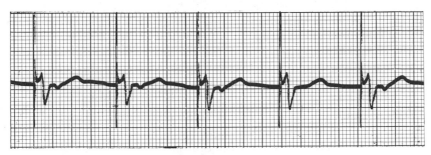

Figure 10-2 Paced ventricular rhythm with retrograde P waves.

Complete the following sentences:

1. Typical features of junctional rhythm include _____ P waves and _____ QRS complexes.

2. During junctional rhythm, an inverted P wave may follow the QRS complex when antegrade conduction to the _____ precedes _____ conduction to the _____ .

3. In Figure 10-3, the R-to-R interval is _____ sec and the heart rate is _____ bpm. A _____ P wave follows each QRS complex. This EKG shows _____ rhythm.

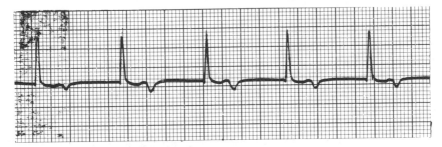

Figure 10-3

4. P waves may not be visible during junctional rhythm when _____ depolarization and _____ depolarization occur simultaneously.

Review.   Retrograde P waves and narrow supraventricular QRS configuration are typical features of junctional rhythm. If antegrade ventricular activation precedes retrograde conduction to the atria, a retrograde P wave follows the QRS. When atrial and ventricular activation are simultaneous, retrograde P waves are obscured by QRS complexes.

In Figure 10-3, the rate of 69 bpm corresponds to an R-to-R interval of 0.88 sec and retrograde P waves confirm the presence of accelerated junctional rhythm.

An electronic pacemaker may establish an artificial ectopic atrial rhythm. In this case, the ectopic focus is a contact point between the pacing electrode and the atrial wall. P waves during atrial pacing are abnormal. Examine Figure 10-4. A pacing artifact is present before each P wave. The PRI and QRS complexes are normal.

An atrial ectopic focus may accelerate to a rapid rate. This form of tachycardia is particularly characteristic of digitalis toxicity associated with hypokalemia. Figure 10-5 shows typical features of this rhythm disorder. P waves are regular, usually at a rate of 140 to 200 bpm. They are clearly separated by a flat segment of the EKG baseline. P wave configuration is usually abnormal. At rapid atrial rates, especially when digitalis toxicity has slowed AV node conduction, some atrial impulses are not conducted to the ventricles. The resulting rhythm is *atrial tachycardia with block*. The AV conduction ratio may vary, leading to an irregular ventricular rate.

During atrial tachycardia with block, P waves are often concealed by larger QRS complexes or T waves. Two methods are commonly useful in searching for concealed P waves: comparing adjacent complexes or using calipers to measure successive P-to-P intervals. The search should begin in leads II and V_1, which ordinarily display P waves most clearly. Occasionally, special leads must be used, including a pervenous electrode advanced into the right atrial chamber to record atrial depolarization.

Figure 10-6 illustrates P wave detection by subtle differences in adjacent complexes. In Figure 10-6(A), a P wave coincides with the T wave of the second complex. This *P on T* causes an apparent increase in T wave amplitude as compared to the next T wave. In Figure 10-6(B), the P wave falls at the end of the QRS complex, causing an apparent increase in QRS duration.

In Figure 10-5, the P-to-P interval is regular. Use calipers set at

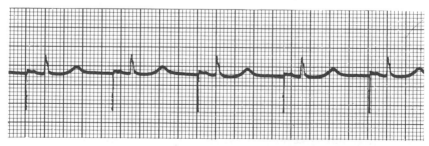

Figure 10-4   Paced atrial rhythm.

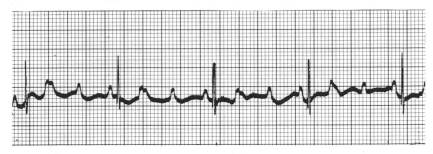

Figure 10-5   Atrial tachycardia with block. Atrial rate is 180 bpm. The AV conduction ratio is 3 : 1.

this interval to time successive intervals and to discover that several P waves are partially hidden by T waves.

An unusual rhythm disorder occurs when impulses form at a rapid rate in several separate atrial foci. This rhythm, called *multifocal atrial tachycardia,* is seen principally in patients with pulmonary failure. P waves are irregular in timing and varied in configuration. PR intervals typically vary. Ventricular rate is usually 120 to 140 bpm. QRS complexes reflect supraventricular origin of depolarization. Examine Figure 10-7. Note the changing P-to-P intervals and different P wave shapes. QRS complexes are totally irregular at a rate near 150 bpm.

Complete the following sentences:

1. A change in P wave configuration may result from either a change in site of origin of _____ depolarization or a change in intraatrial _____ .

2. _____ _____ _____ is characterized by rapid, irregular P waves of varying configuration.

3. During _____ _____ with block, often a

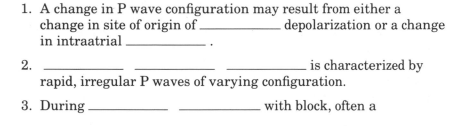

Figure 10-6   P waves obscured by (A) T wave or (B) QRS complex.

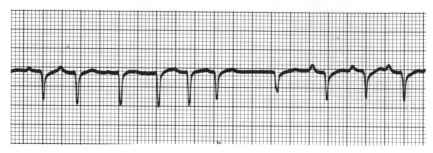

Figure 10-7 Multifocal atrial tachycardia. P waves vary in shape. Their timing is rapid and irregular. QRS complexes show narrow supraventricular configuration.

manifestation of _____ toxicity, adjacent P waves are distinctly separated by a segment of the _____ and the _____ conduction ratio may change frequently.

Review. P wave configuration may change because of ectopic origin of atrial depolarization or because of a change in intraatrial conduction when depolarization originates in the SA node. Multifocal atrial tachycardia results in rapid P waves of differing shape. Atrial tachycardia with block may be due to digitalis toxicity; P waves are separated by segments of the EKG baseline and AV conduction may vary.

Lesson 11

Atrial Tachyarrhythmias

Lesson 11 concerns EKG waves of atrial origin during three common disorders: atrial flutter (AFl), atrial fibrillation (AF), and paroxysmal supraventricular tachycardia (PSVT). These ectopic rhythms, characterized by rapid abnormal atrial depolarization, arise at sites above the His bundle and its branches. In Lesson 10, you learned about ectopic supraventricular impulse formation in cells that depolarize automatically. In contrast, the rhythm disorders discussed in Lesson 11 are typically caused by another form of abnormal origin of depolarization—reentry.

Reentry depends on repeated flow of depolarization around a conduction circuit. Anatomically, the reentry circuit may be localized to a small area involving only short segments of interconnected fibers. Other circuits may include long conduction tracts within the atria and ventricles. From the reentry circuit, depolarization spreads to the heart chambers. The process may be limited to a single cycle, manifested as a premature ectopic beat. If reentry continues for a short series of cycles, the result is a salvo of ectopic beats. Persistent reentry causes a sustained tachyarrhythmia.

Examine Figure 11-1(A), which diagrams normal depolarization of interconnected fibers, a structural pattern that occurs abundantly throughout the heart. Depolarization entering the circuit at point X will be conducted symmetrically through both branches of the circuit and will terminate at point Y. A region of slow conduction in one branch of the circuit, such as in zone Z of Figure 11-1(B), provides a setting for reentry. Depolarization may spread through the more rapid conduction

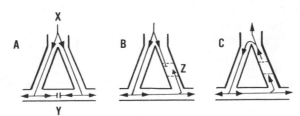

Figure 11-1 Mechanism of reentry.

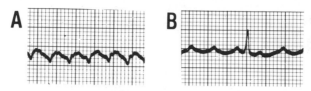

Figure 11-2 Configuration of AFl waves at rates of (A) 300 and (B) 250 bpm.

pathway of the circuit and cross zone Z in a retrograde direction. It may then reenter the circuit and spread from it to the heart through all available pathways [Figure 11-1(C)]. Once initiated, the process may continue indefinitely. Each depolarization of an atrial reentrant focus will spread to the atria and result in an abnormal atrial EKG wave.

AFl is a common reentrant arrhythmia characterized by regular, well-organized atrial depolarization, usually at a rate between 240 and 360 bpm. Figure 11-2 illustrates typical AFl waves (f waves). Their configuration is uniform and often somewhat peaked or "saw-toothed." The EKG during AFl typically shows continuous movement of the baseline; flat baseline segments are not present between adjacent waves.

During AFl, the AV node does not conduct every atrial impulse. Common AV conduction ratios are 2:1 and 4:1. The conduction ratio may be unstable, and the ventricular rate then becomes irregular. When the conduction ratio is 2:1, the diagnosis of AFl may be unclear because a QRS complex may obscure every second flutter wave. Examine Figure 11-3(A). Flutter waves are present at a regular rate of

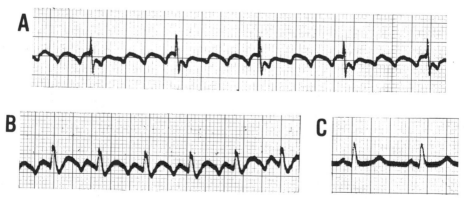

Figure 11-3 AFl with (A) 4:1 AV conduction and (B) 2:1 AV conduction.

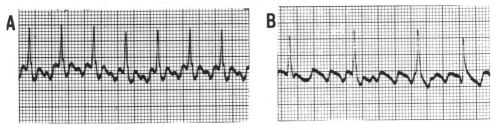

Figure 11-4 AFl (A) before and (B) after CSP.

270 bpm. The 4 : 1 AV conduction ratio is stable, resulting in a regular ventricular rate of 68 bpm. Figure 11-3(B) shows AFl with 2 : 1 AV conduction. A QRS complex obscures every second flutter wave. Compare these QRS complexes to those shown in Figure 11-3(C), recorded after restoration of sinus rhythm. Note that the hidden flutter waves can be identified by this comparison because they alter QRS complex configuration.

AFl with 2 : 1 AV conduction is a common clinical problem and should be considered whenever the EKG shows a regular tachycardia near 150 bpm with supraventricular QRS complexes. Pressure on the carotid sinus, or other methods of vagal stimulation, may clarify the diagnosis. Vagal stimulation slows AV node conduction and may decrease the AV conduction ratio, exposing previously hidden flutter waves. Examine Figure 11-4. In this illustration, carotid sinus pressure (CSP) changes the AV conduction ratio from 2 : 1 to 4 : 1, and flutter waves become apparent.

Complete the following sentences:

1. The electrophysiologic basis for typical AFl is _____ ; atrial rate exceeds _____ bpm.

2. In Figure 11-5, the atrial rate is _____ bpm. The ventricular rate is _____ bpm; the ventricular rhythm is irregular because of a changing _____ _____ ratio.

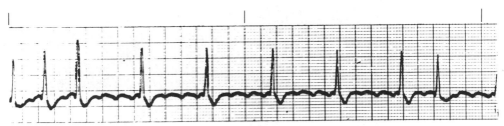

Figure 11-5

Review. Reentry within an atrial ectopic circuit is the basis for AFl and leads to atrial rates greater than 240 bpm. The atrial rate in Figure 11-5 is 300 bpm. An unstable AV conduction ratio is responsible for an irregular ventricular rhythm at a rate of 90 bpm, which must be estimated by a 6-sec count of QRS complexes. Begin this count with the QRS complex following the beat that marks the start of the counting interval.

AF, the most common atrial tachyarrhythmia, causes rapid, totally irregular atrial EKG waves of varying configuration. Because separate fibrillation waves are not clearly delineated, their rate in beats per minute is usually indeterminate. They represent disorganized, multifocal atrial reentry. Many of the rapid atrial impulses that enter the AV node are not conducted to the ventricles. The resulting ventricular rhythm is totally irregular. The ventricular rate depends on AV node function; it is usually 140 to 180 bpm before treatment. Elderly patients tend to have a slower ventricular response to AF.

Figure 11-6 illustrates atrial wave patterns during AF. The fibrillation waves in Figure 11-6(A) are large, or coarse. In Figure 11-6(B), AF waves are small and not clearly evident. When atrial waves are not present, an irregular ventricular rate with supraventricular QRS complexes may be the only EKG manifestation of AF. Occasionally, as in Figure 11-6(C), AF waves may change transiently to a more organized and regular pattern sometimes referred to as atrial flutter-fibrillation.

PSVT, also referred to as *paroxysmal atrial tachycardia* (PAT), is another common supraventricular rhythm disorder caused by reentry. It may occur in young patients who have no other evidence of heart

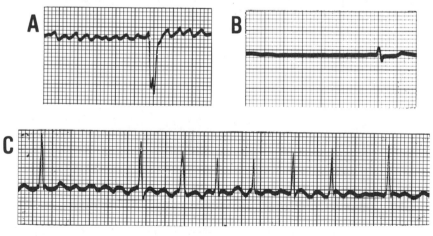

Figure 11-6 AF waves.

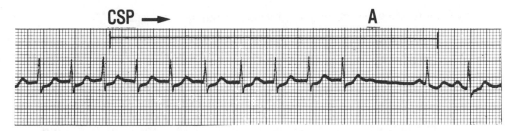

Figure 11-7 PSVT (AV nodal reentrant tachycardia) with conversion to normal sinus rhythm after CSP.

disease. Its onset is abrupt, typically triggered by a premature atrial beat. QRS complexes are precisely regular at a rate between 140 and 220 bpm. Reentry in a circuit within the AV node is the usual basis for PSVT. From this focus, depolarization may spread retrograde to the atria. Atrial waves are commonly absent during PSVT because atrial and ventricular depolarization occur simultaneously.

Examine Figure 11-7, an example of PSVT. During the tachycardia, P waves are not evident. Use calipers to show that the ventricular rhythm is regular at a rate of 140 bpm. Narrow supraventricular QRS complexes are present. At point A, the tachycardia ceases. After a pause, sinus rhythm resumes.

Remember that AFl with 2 : 1 conduction is another possible cause of a rapid, regular supraventricular rhythm at a ventricular rate of 140 bpm. In AFl, the vagal effect of CSP reduces AV conduction and exposes hidden f waves. As Figure 11-7 illustrates, the effect of CSP on PSVT is quite different. Vagal stimulation will often interrupt an AV nodal reentrant circuit and terminate PSVT.

Complete the following sentences:

1. Characteristics of AF include absence of _____ waves, totally _____ ventricular rhythm and _____ QRS configuration as seen when origin of depolarization is above the His bundle.

2. The ladder diagram in Figure 11-8 initially shows _____ rhythm, then a premature atrial beat that initiates _____ within the AV node.

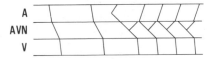

Figure 11-8

3. Of the three common types of regular supraventricular tachycardia (SVT), CSP may terminate _____ , decrease the AV conduction ratio during _____ , or cause transient gradual slowing of heart rate during ST.

Review.   During AF, P waves are absent and supraventricular QRS complexes are totally irregular. Figure 11-8 diagrams normal sinus rhythm followed by a premature atrial beat that initiates AV nodal reentry. CSP may terminate PSVT or slow the ventricular rate during AFl.

Lesson 12

Abnormal P Waves of Atrial Enlargement

In Lessons 10 and 11, you learned about abnormal atrial waves related to origin of depolarization in atrial ectopic foci that are the site of automatic impulse formation or of reentry. A different category of abnormal atrial waves occurs during normal sinus rhythm as a result of right atrial or left atrial enlargement. These abnormalities may be associated with many different forms of heart disease, especially valvular disease, congenital heart disease, or congestive heart failure. They may be diagnostic clues or may provide indirect information about the degree of severity of an underlying disease.

Atrial enlargement is often a relatively complex pathophysiologic state. Either atrium, or both together, may be altered by chronic work overloads. The work load may result because the atrium must pump excessive amounts of blood (volume overload) or because it must pump at abnormally high pressure to expel blood through a stenotic valve or into a stiff ventricle that is resistant to filling (pressure overload). An atrium often must respond simultaneously to both volume and pressure overloads. Depending on the type, severity, and duration of overload, the atrium may dilate, thicken, or both. Fibrosis and other degenerative changes may occur in the atrial wall. In view of this pathophysiologic complexity, it is not surprising that EKG abnormalities associated with atrial enlargement may at times be at variance with radiographic or ultrasound evidence of atrial dilatation.

In Lesson 5, you learned that normal P waves reflect the sequence of atrial depolarization as it spreads from the SA node to the right atrium and then to the left atrium. This sequence is especially well displayed in lead V_1, where the normal P wave has a negative left atrial component. Left atrial enlargement (LAE) typically delays the left atrial P wave component and increases its magnitude. The terminal negative P wave component in lead V_1 then becomes more than 1.0 mm (0.04 sec) wide and more than 1.0 mm (0.1 mV) deep. In lead II, LAE widens the P wave to a duration of 0.12 sec or more, and the P wave acquires a prominent notch, or double hump. The two humps, corresponding to right atrial and delayed left atrial depolarization, are at least 0.04 sec apart.

Examine Figure 12-1. The normal P wave, Figure 12-1(A), is only slightly notched in lead II; and the dimensions of its terminal component in lead V_1 are less than 1.0×1.0 mm. The P wave in Figure 12-1(B) shows moderate abnormalities of LAE. The left atrial component is enlarged in V_1 and the notched P wave in lead II is 0.14 sec wide. The P wave in Figure 12-1(C) shows more advanced evidence of LAE. Figure 12-1(D) shows an atypical pattern, with marked prolongation of P wave duration to 0.16 sec. This abnormality may reflect an interatrial conduction delay due to dysfunction of interatrial conduction fibers, rather than to LAE.

Right atrial enlargement (RAE) increases P wave amplitude. It does not delay left atrial depolarization and P wave duration remains normal. The P wave abnormality of RAE is most prominent in the inferior lead group of the frontal plane, leads II, III, and aVF. In these leads, P waves typically become peaked and exceed 2.5 to 3.0 mm in height at standard calibration (1 mV = 10 mm). In lead V_1, the initial P wave component corresponding to right atrial depolarization may be enlarged.

Examine Figure 12-2. The normal P wave, Figure 12-2(A), is 2.0 mm in height in lead III. The P wave in Figure 12-2(B), is 3.5 mm high and 0.8 sec in duration. It has a peaked configuration typical of RAE. The right atrial component of the P wave in lead V_1 is also peaked and unusually prominent. The P wave in Figure 12-2(C) shows evidence of combined RAE and LAE. The P wave is wide, and both its initial and terminal components are enlarged in lead V_1.

Criteria for atrial enlargement should not be rigidly applied in routine EKG interpretation. For many normal subjects, the terminal P wave component in lead V_1 may be slightly greater than 1.0 mm deep and more than 1.0 mm wide. This minor abnormality may be considered innocuous or borderline. The reliability of inferences based on EKG waves will commonly depend on the degree of abnormality, the number

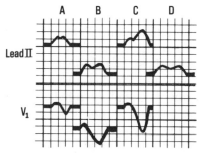

Figure 12-1 P wave abnormalities due to (B and C) left atrial enlargement and (D) interatrial conduction delay.

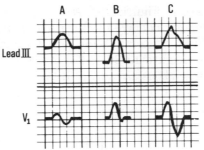

Figure 12-2 P wave abnormalities due to (B) RAE and (C) biatrial enlargement.

of leads that show the abnormality, and the likelihood based on other information that an individual patient will in fact have the anatomic finding suggested by the EKG wave pattern.

Complete the following sentences:

1. In Figure 12-3(A), P wave duration is _____ sec in lead II and its peaks are _____ sec apart, indicating delayed depolarization of the _____ _____ .

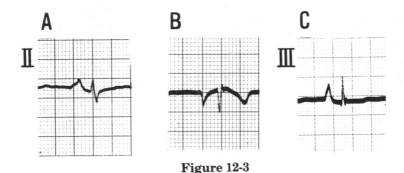

Figure 12-3

2. The terminal P wave component in Figure 12-3(B) is _____ mm wide and _____ mm deep, a finding in lead _____ that suggests _____ atrial enlargement.

3. The P wave in Figure 12-3(C) is _____ mm tall and _____ sec in duration. This finding in the _____ lead group suggests _____ _____ enlargement.

Review.   The P wave in Figure 12-3(A) is 0.16 sec wide, with peaks 0.04 sec apart, as seen with delayed left atrial depolarization. The V_1 P wave of Figure 12-3(B) is 2.0 mm wide and 3.0 mm deep, suggesting LAE. The P wave in Figure 12-3(C), 3.0 mm tall and 0.10 sec wide, occurs in the inferior leads as a result of RAE.

3 | Abnormal QRS Complexes

Lesson 13

Bundle Branch Block and Other Intraventricular Conduction Delays

As you have learned, normal function of specialized rapid conduction fibers in the His–Purkinje system is essential for rapid ventricular depolarization and normal QRS duration of 0.10 sec or less. When a total conduction block occurs in the proximal portion of the RBB or LBB, complete ventricular depolarization requires 0.12 sec or more. This degree of QRS complex widening is the first criterion for diagnosis of complete bundle branch block (BBB). Less frequently, the QRS shows a BBB pattern with QRS width of 0.10 to 0.12 sec, a finding termed *incomplete BBB*. Complete or incomplete BBB may occur in a wide variety of heart diseases that enhance fibrotic degeneration of the conduction system. BBB commonly accompanies hypertensive heart disease, coronary artery disease, and aortic valve disease. It may also occur in the absence of other manifestations of heart disease, especially in elderly persons. In rare instances, BBB is present in young subjects who are otherwise well. The conduction defect may be permanent or intermittent.

Typical uncomplicated right bundle branch block (RBBB) causes an easily recognized QRS abnormality. Remember that the first phase of ventricular activation is septal depolarization from fibers of the *left* bundle branch. RBBB does not alter this initial QRS force. Its principal effect is to delay depolarization of right ventricular zones located at a distance from the ventricular septum. The QRS complex widens because delayed right ventricular forces are added to it.

Examine Figure 13-1 closely. It illustrates typical QRS complex configuration in leads I and V_1 before [Figure 13-1(A)] and after [Figure 13-1(B)] RBBB. Delayed RV forces are directed anteriorly and to the right. These forces are represented in V_1 by a wide prominent R' wave that is commonly notched and in lead I by a wide S wave. QRS duration widens to 0.12 sec. Figure 13-1(C) illustrates incomplete RBBB with delayed right ventricular forces and QRS width 0.11 sec.

Left bundle branch block (LBBB), in contrast, delays all phases of left ventricular depolarization. The typical result is a diffusely widened and notched R wave in leads I and V_6. Figure 13-2 illustrates this

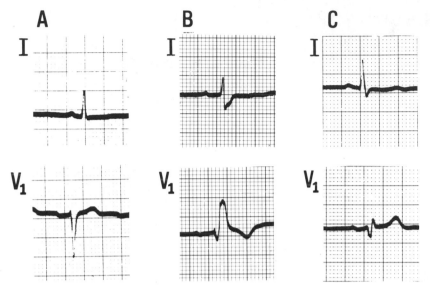

Figure 13-1 QRS effects of (B) complete RBBB and (C) incomplete RBBB.

abnormality. Note that before LBBB [Figure 13-2(A)], a small Q wave in lead V_6 and an R wave in V_1 display normal initial septal depolarization. These waves are commonly lost when LBBB develops.

Complete the following sentences:

1. _____ BBB changes the pattern of septal depolarization, commonly with loss of _____ waves in V_1.

2. Figure 13-3 illustrates a sequence of three major ventricular depolarization forces in the horizontal plane. The direction of terminal force C is _____ and _____ , as seen when _____ is present.

3. BBB can be diagnosed only when origin of depolarization is _____ .

Review. Septal r waves in V_1 are commonly lost because of LBBB. Anterior and rightward terminal force C of Figure 13-3 is typical of delayed right ventricular forces due to RBBB. Only when origin of depolarization is supraventricular can BBB be recognized.

An important form of temporary BBB may appear during supraventricular tachyarrhythmias or premature beats. This abnormality is termed *aberrant ventricular conduction* (AVC) to distinguish it from other forms of BBB. AVC usually results in a RBBB pattern, although typical LBBB may also occur. Examine Figure 13-4. Atrial

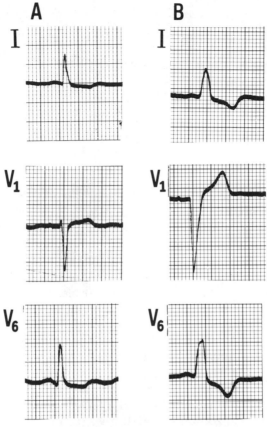

Figure 13-2 QRS effects of LBBB.

fibrillation is the underlying rhythm disorder, initially with a normal QRS complex. The wide QRS complexes due to AVC show a RBBB pattern, without change in initial QRS forces.

QRS duration may be prolonged for reasons other than BBB. When conduction is uniformly slowed in His–Purkinje fibers, the QRS complex widens symmetrically without a major change in configuration.

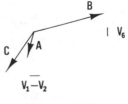

Figure 13-3

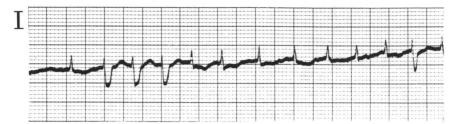

Figure 13-4   AF (lead I) with intermittent wide QRS complexes due to AVC.

This pattern of nonspecific intraventricular conduction delay (IVCD) may be caused by drugs or severe hyperkalemia, as illustrated in Figure 13-5(A). Figure 13-5(B) shows another form of QRS widening with a bizarre configuration that may accompany diseased ventricular muscle.

Another category of ventricular conduction abnormality may result from fibrosis or other disorders involving either of the two principal divisions, or fascicles, of the LBB. Fascicular block is also referred to as hemiblock. Because alternative conduction pathways are abundant in the left ventricle, fascicular block does not cause a major ventricular depolarization delay. The QRS duration is not greater than 0.10 sec. Fascicular block alters the sequence of left ventricular depolarization and shifts the frontal plane QRS axis. With typical block in the anterior fascicle of the LAFB, left axis deviation between −45 and −90° is present. Initial QRS forces are directed inferiorly and are displayed as a small r wave in lead III and by small q waves in leads I and aVL. An associated shift of QRS forces in the horizontal plane commonly results in clockwise rotation or poor R wave progression in the precordial leads. Block of the posterior fascicle (LPFB) is relatively rare. Its principal manifestation is right axis deviation with an initial R wave in leads I and aVL.

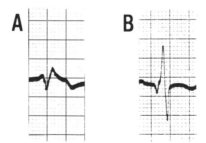

Figure 13-5   Wide QRS complexes due to (A) hyperkalemia and (B) cardiomyopathy.

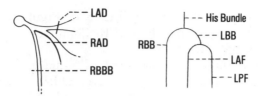

Figure 13-6 Diagrammatic representation of a trifascicular ventricular conduction system and consequences of fascicular block.

Figure 13-6 illustrates the concept of a trifascicular ventricular conduction system, indicating that the RBB and the two fascicles of the LBB form parallel pathways for conduction of supraventricular impulses to the ventricles. Although the actual branching pattern of the LBB is more complex than implied by this diagram, the concept is a useful model with important implications. Fibrosis and other disorders of the ventricular conduction system tend to involve all pathways, although their vulnerability and degree of involvement vary considerably. Dual pathway, or bifascicular, block leads to a combination of the

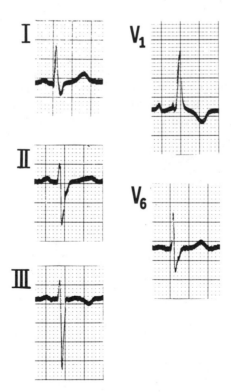

Figure 13-7 Bifascicular block (LAFB and RBBB).

individual EKG abnormalities indicated in Figure 13-6, most commonly RBBB with LAD due to LAFB. Complete trifascicular block interrupts AV conduction entirely.

Figure 13-7 illustrates combined LAFB and RBBB. LAFB causes LAD, with negative QRS in lead II. Additional RBBB does not alter the initial QRS forces, but prolongs QRS duration to 0.12 sec with a wide S wave present in lead I.

Complete the following sentences:

1. An elderly patient's EKG shows LAFB, with QRS axis between _____ and _____ ° and a small _____ wave in aVL. A subsequent tracing shows QRS duration 0.12 sec and a wide, notched R wave in lead I, indicating that _____ has developed.

2. AVC may occur during _____ tachyarrhythmias, usually causing _____ bundle branch block with a wide R′ wave in lead _____ .

3. Three broad categories of wide QRS complexes greater than 0.12 sec in duration are _____   _____ block, _____   _____ conduction, and nonspecific _____   _____ delay.

Review. QRS axis is between −45 and −90°, and a small q wave is present in aVL as the result of LAFB, which may progress to LBBB. AVC during atrial tachyarrhythmias usually mimics RBBB, with wide R′ in V_1. BBB, AVC, and IVCD are three categories of wide QRS complexes.

Lesson 14

Ventricular Ectopic Depolarization / Fusion Beats

Normal depolarization sequence of a cardiac chamber depends on normal origin of depolarization and on normally functioning conduction pathways. In Lesson 13, you saw the consequences of disturbed conduction within the His–Purkinje system, leading to BBB and related defects that delay the spread of depolarization. Lesson 14 discusses delayed spread of ventricular depolarization due to origin of depolarization in an ectopic ventricular focus. Ventricular ectopic impulse formation occurs in both healthy hearts and many disease states. For CAD patients with poor LV pump function and in other advanced disease states, ventricular ectopy may be life threatening. In many other settings, ventricular ectopic beats are innocuous.

The mechanisms of ectopic ventricular activity correspond to atrial ectopic mechanisms discussed in Lessons 10 and 11: automaticity and reentry. An ectopic focus may appear in the wall of either ventricle or in the ventricular septum. From this focus, depolarization spreads throughout the ventricles by all available pathways, including neighboring branches of the His–Purkinje system. It also spreads retrograde to the AV node and at times through the node to the atrium. The principal EKG manifestation of this disordered spread of depolarization is readily predicted: the QRS complex is deformed and abnormally wide, typically with duration of 0.12 sec or greater.

Figure 14-1 illustrates a ventricular ectopic focus in the LV wall, with spread of depolarization from this site as shown by arrows. Arrow A represents spread of depolarization along the LV aspect of the ventricular septum, where it enters central conduction fibers and travels retrograde to the AV node (arrow B). Arrow C indicates spread of depolarization toward the RV, where it enters the distal fibers of the RBB and spreads to the remaining RV wall. Delayed RV depolarization is also a feature of RBBB, and QRS complexes originating in a LV ectopic focus generally have RBBB configuration as shown in Figure 14-1. Conversely, RV ectopy results in a QRS pattern resembling LBBB.

Examine Figure 14-2. Sinus rhythm is present. Most of the com-

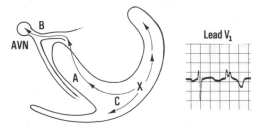

Figure 14-1 Ventricular depolarization from an LV ectopic focus (X).

plexes show a normal relationship between P waves and QRS complexes. Two premature complexes are present, each with QRS duration greater than 0.12 sec. The wide QRS complexes have quite different patterns, implying that they originate from different sites in the ventricles. Premature ventricular ectopic beats of varying configuration are commonly described as *multifocal*.

In Figure 14-3 a series of wide QRS beats is present at a rate of 150 bpm, an example of ventricular tachycardia. This rhythm ordinarily results from repetitive reentry in a ventricular ectopic focus.

Figure 14-4 shows irregular waves of varying configuration, an example of ventricular fibrillation, the result of rapid ventricular activity with totally disorganized spread of depolarization.

Examine Figure 14-5. The first two cycles of this lead V_1 rhythm strip show sinus rhythm at 95 bpm with narrow QRS complexes, but with marked prolongation of the QT interval. The third beat is premature and initiates an unusual type of reentrant multiform ventricular tachycardia, referred to as *torsades de pointes* (twisting of the points) because groups of the wide QRS complexes point alternately up or down.

Complete the following sentences:

1. Figure 14-6 shows a paced ventricular beat with a
   wide _____ wave in lead I, resembling _____ BBB

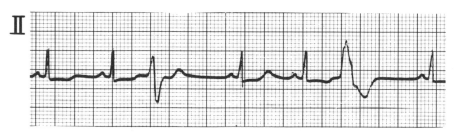

Figure 14-2 Ectopic ventricular depolarization from two foci.

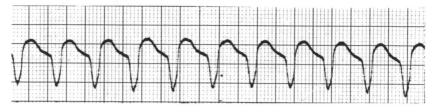

Figure 14-3   Ventricular tachycardia.

and suggesting that the pacing electrode is in contact with the _____ ventricle.

2. QRS complexes associated with ventricular ectopy are usually at least _____ sec in duration because _____ of a part of the ventricle is delayed.

Review.   The RBBB pattern in Figure 14-6, with a wide S wave in lead I, indicates LV pacing. Delayed ventricular depolarization widens ectopic QRS complexes to more than 0.12 sec.

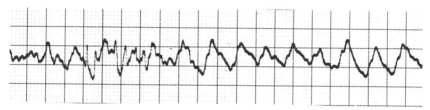

Figure 14-4   Ventricular fibrillation.

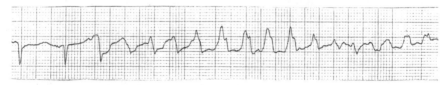

Figure 14-5   Multiform ventricular tachycardia *torsades de pointes*.

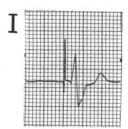

Figure 14-6

In Lesson 1, you learned that ventricular fibers in the His–Purkinje network can become automatic pacing cells, capable of spontaneous depolarization, typically at a rate of 35 bpm. When more rapid supraventricular pacing cells are not functioning, the ventricular pacing fibers capture heart rhythm, establishing a slow *idioventricular escape rhythm*. These fibers may also accelerate to rates much faster than 35 bpm and may then compete with normal supraventricular pacemakers.

At times, ventricular depolarization may originate simultaneously from two separate points. The result is a *fusion beat*. Figure 14-7 illustrates this phenomenon. The diagram indicates that part of the ventricles, marked by striations, is depolarized through the normal supraventricular pathway, A. The remaining ventricle is activated at the same time from an ectopic ventricular focus, X. On the EKG strip, note that the fusion complex, F, has an intermediate form, sharing features of the normal QRS, A, and of the ectopic QRS, X.

Examine Figure 14-8, an example of accelerated idioventricular rhythm at a rate of 48 bpm that competes with a slow sinus rhythm. AV dissociation is present initially when ventricular depolarization originates from an ectopic focus and atrial depolarization originates from the SA node. The third QRS complex is a fusion beat that occurs when a supraventricular impulse reaches the ventricles after they have been partially depolarized from the idioventricular pacing focus.

Figure 14-9 illustrates an unusual type of ventricular fusion beat that may occur when an atrial depolarization reaches the ventricles through two separate conduction pathways, the normal His bundle (A) and an abnormal path between atria and ventricles, the bundle of Kent (B). The Kent bundle bypasses the AV node; conduction through this pathway is not delayed. Kent bundle depolarization reaches the ventricles early and captures a segment of the ventricular wall, a form of "preexcitation." The QRS complex that results is abnormally wide because an early component, the delta wave, has been added to it. The configuration of the delta wave depends on the anatomic location of the Kent bundle. The delta wave is superimposed on the PR interval, which appears shortened. The short PR interval, wide QRS complex, and delta wave characterize the Wolff-Parkinson-White (WPW) syndrome.

The following list summarizes frequent or important causes of wide QRS complexes:

1. BBB.
2. Ventricular ectopic origin of depolarization.
3. AVC.
4. WPW syndrome.
5. Nonspecific intraventricular conduction delay.

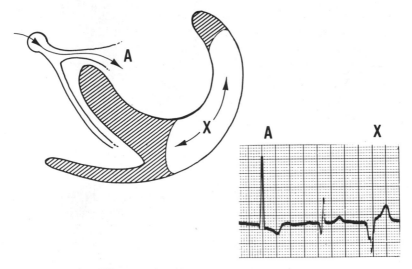

Figure 14-7 Ventricular fusion beat.

Complete the following sentences:

1. Accelerated idioventricular rhythm results in a _____ beat when the ventricle is partially depolarized by an ectopic focus, whereas the remaining ventricle is depolarized by a _____ impulse.

2. When an accelerated automatic focus in the RV captures ventricular rhythm, QRS complexes will have a wide, notched R wave in leads _____ and _____ , as seen with _____ BBB.

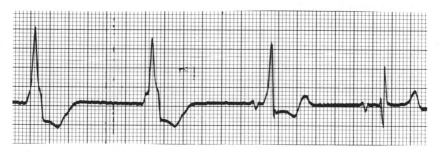

Figure 14-8 Idioventricular rhythm with fusion beat.

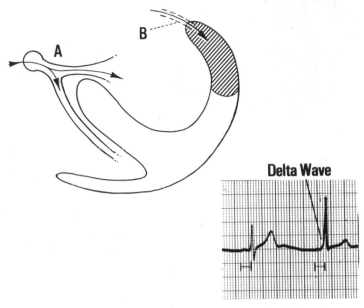

Delta Wave

Figure 14-9 Ventricular fusion beat due to AV bypass tract (WPW syndrome).

3. When an atrial depolarization reaches the ventricle through two separate AV conduction pathways, a _____ wave appears, shortening the _____ interval and widening the _____ .

Review. A fusion beat results when an ectopic automatic focus and a supraventricular impulse simultaneously participate in ventricular depolarization. An RV focus typically results in a LBBB pattern with wide R waves in leads I and V$_6$. Partial early ventricular depolarization through an abnormal pathway results in a delta wave, short PRI, and wide QRS complex.

Lesson 15

QRS Abnormalities Due to Ventricular Hypertrophy

The complex anatomic pathology and electrophysiology of atrial enlargement discussed in Lesson 12 have even more complex parallels related to ventricular hypertrophy and its diagnosis from the EKG. Either ventricle, or both together, may thicken or dilate in response to pressure or volume overloads of varying severity and duration. A ventricle may hypertrophy symmetrically or asymmetrically, even in the absence of work overload. Conduction abnormalities, including BBB, are common in a thickened ventricle. It is essential to understand that ventricular hypertrophy is not an easily defined entity. An anatomic definition based on ventricular weight adjusted for body weight or body surface area is of limited value. For clinical purposes, ventricular hypertrophy should be considered a spectrum of abnormalities. In evaluation of an individual patient, the 12-lead EKG contributes valuable, but not definitive, evidence to a profile of findings that relate to ventricular chamber size.

Left ventricular hypertrophy (LVH) has two principal effects on the QRS complex: increase in amplitude and increase in duration. Either or both of these abnormalities may be present. A secondary effect is leftward displacement of the QRS axis. QRS forces may also be displaced posteriorly, resulting in poor R wave progression in the precordial leads.

High QRS voltage is usually most prominent in the chest leads, but at times may be evident only in the limb leads. Routine voltage measurements are made for the R wave in V_5 or V_6, whichever is larger; for the larger S wave in V_1 or V_2; and for the largest R or S wave in lead I or III. As you learned in Lesson 6, R or S wave voltage in a chest lead should not exceed 30 mm at standard calibration (1 mV = 10 mm) except in young patients. The sum of the S wave in V_1 or V_2 and the R wave in V_5 or V_6 should not exceed 40 mm. The R or S wave in lead I or III should not exceed 20 mm. Other voltage criteria for LVH have been proposed and may be applied for individuals who have other evidence or high risk for this abnormality; for example, S wave V_{1-2} plus R wave V_{5-6} greater than 35 mm, or R wave aVL greater than 11 mm.

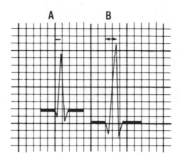

Figure 15-1 Intrinsicoid deflection (ID); (A) normal ID = 0.03 sec and (B) delayed ID = 0.06 sec.

Widening of the QRS complex due to LVH may reflect increased activation time for thickened muscle mass or an associated conduction system dysfunction. Usually, the QRS duration does not exceed 0.12 sec. Widening is evident in the initial QRS forces, and at times it is helpful to determine the intrinsicoid deflection, as illustrated in Figure 15-1. Select a lead with tall R waves, usually V_6 or lead I, and measure the time interval from onset of the QRS complex to the end of the R wave peak. This interval should not exceed 0.045 sec.

Complete the following sentences:

1. Figure 15-2 shows a QRS complex from the EKG of a 25-year-old athlete, with an R wave of _____ mm. The intrinsicoid deflection is _____ sec. You conclude that this complex is _____ for a young person.

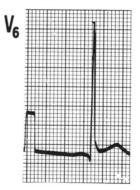

Figure 15-2

2. Figure 15-3 shows a lead I QRS complex with voltage of _____ mm and QRS width of _____ sec. You conclude that this patient has _____ .

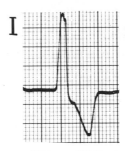

Figure 15-3

Review. V_6 R wave amplitude for the 25-year-old patient is 34 mm. Note that the calibration artifact indicates standard calibration, or 1 mV = 10 mm. The intrinsicoid deflection is 0.04 sec. These findings are normal at age 25. In Figure 15-3, the R wave is 21 mm and QRS duration is 0.16 sec. This patient has LBBB. The conduction abnormality may account for high QRS voltage and LVH cannot be diagnosed reliably when LBBB is present.

Right ventricular hypertrophy (RVH) is uncommon and, in part for this reason, is a source of diagnostic errors in EKG interpretation. RVH has two principal effects on the QRS complex: RAD and prominent R waves in V_1. In lead V_1 normal R wave amplitude should not exceed S wave amplitude; the R-to-S ratio is normally less than 1. Configuration of the lead V_1 complex has a useful correlation with the type of right ventricular work overload. Major pressure overload, as seen with pulmonic valve stenosis or severe pulmonary hypertension, causes generalized RV hypertrophy and lead V_1 typically shows a qR configuration, illustrated in Figure 15-4(B). Volume overload, as seen with atrial septal defect, leads to major hypertrophy of the RV outflow tract, the last segment of the ventricle to depolarize. Outflow tract hypertrophy is associated with an rSR' configuration as shown in Figure 15-4(C).

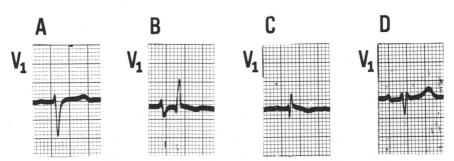

Figure 15-4 QRS effects of RVH (B, C) and incomplete RBBB (D) in lead V_1 compared to normal complex (A).

Incomplete RBBB may result in a similar configuration with QRS duration between 0.10 and 0.12 sec, as in Figure 15-4(D). A small r' wave in lead V_1 may occur in normal young people.

In older patients, especially in the presence of pulmonary emphysema, EKG evidence of RVH may be subtle or atypical. Emphysema may cause downward displacement or rotation of the heart and may alter electrical conductance within the chest. As a result, QRS voltage may be abnormally low. In patients with emphysema, RAD and marked clockwise rotation suggests RVH.

Biventricular hypertrophy is another source of diagnostic ambiguity. The EKG may show only minor abnormalities, or a combination of criteria such as RAD with voltage evidence for LVH.

Complete the following sentences:

1. Figure 15-5 shows an abnormal _____ wave in lead V_1 and a corresponding prominent _____ wave in lead V_6. P wave configuration in V_1 suggests _____ .

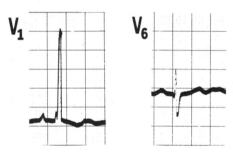

Figure 15-5

2. In Figure 15-6, the letter notation describing the QRS complex configuration in lead V_1 is _____ . QRS duration is _____ sec. This patient has _____ .

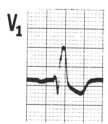

Figure 15-6

Review.   The tall R wave in lead V_1 of Figure 15-5 is abnormal. The corresponding S wave in lead V_6 is large and helps to confirm the EKG diagnosis of RVH when QRS duration is normal, 0.08 sec. The enlarged initial P wave component in V_1 is evidence for right atrial enlargement. The rSR' QRS complex in Figure 15-6 has a duration of 0.16 sec, typical of RBBB.

Lesson 16

QRS Abnormalities Due to Myocardial Infarction

Myocardial infarction, like ventricular hypertrophy, has a wide spectrum of clinical, electrocardiographic, and pathologic features. EKG manifestations generally reflect the stage of infarction, its size, and its anatomic site within the LV. A typical pattern of acute infarction that shows an expected sequence of evolutional changes on a series of tracings has high diagnostic reliability. ST segment and T wave abnormalities of diagnostic importance regularly accompany QRS changes. Conditions other than infarction may mimic EKG infarction patterns, and coexisting abnormalities due to LVH, LBBB, or multiple infarctions may obscure the diagnosis. A normal EKG does not exclude infarction, either acute or old.

The distinctive QRS abnormality of myocardial infarction involves initial QRS forces in lead groups anatomically related to the involved LV segment. Figure 16-1 illustrates the effect of inferior wall infarction. Before infarction [Figure 16-1(A)], oppositely directed forces from the inferior wall and anterolateral wall tend to cancel. After infarction [Figure 16-1(B)], inferior wall forces are diminished and delayed. An unopposed anterolateral force, directed away from the infarction site, is represented by a wide Q wave in the inferior lead group. Q wave evidence of infarction typically appears within hours of onset of the infarction syndrome, but may be delayed for a day or more. As the infarction pattern evolves on serial tracings, Q waves increase in width and amplitude. After weeks or months, Q waves may become smaller or disappear.

Small Q waves are commonly a normal finding in inferior leads III and aVF, or in anterolateral leads aVL, I and V_{5-6}. Normal Q waves generally do not exceed 0.02 sec in duration, or 0.03 sec in lead III, and their amplitude is less than one-third of R wave amplitude in the same lead. Q wave width is the most important criterion for abnormality. Q waves of 0.04 sec duration require explanation. Interpretation of this finding will depend on the clinical setting, the degree of abnormality, the presence of other EKG abnormalities, and the number of adjacent leads that display Q waves.

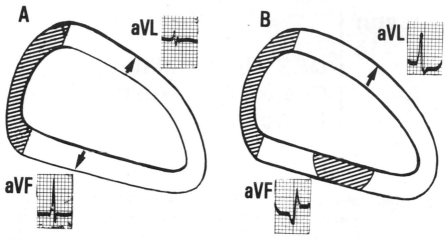

Figure 16-1 QRS effects of inferior wall myocardial infarctions: (A) before infarction and (B) after infarction.

Figure 16-2 illustrates abnormal Q waves due to disorders other than myocardial infarction. In Figure 16-2(A), the lead I complex shows a wide QS wave in a 28-year-old patient with myocardial disease associated with polymyositis. In Figure 16-2(B), the Q wave in lead III is 0.4 seconds wide. Note the delta wave that shortens the PR interval of the lead I complex in the same patient. The lead III Q wave is due to the WPW syndrome and is reciprocally related to the lead I delta wave. These "pseudoinfarction" patterns, although relatively uncommon,

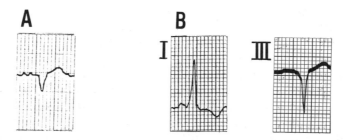

Figure 16-2 Abnormal Q waves in (A) cardiomyopathy and in (B) WPW syndrome.

limit the reliability of diagnosis of myocardial infarction on Q wave criteria alone.

1. Figure 16-3 shows a lead I complex with a Q wave duration of _____ sec. This patient's EKG may also show Q waves in leads _____ and _____ as a result of an old _____ myocardial infarction.

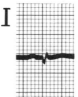

Figure 16-3

2. In Figure 16-4, lead III complexes on serial tracings indicate evolution of acute _____ myocardial infarction.

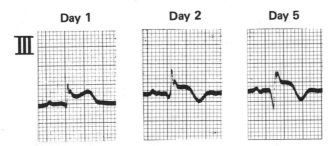

Figure 16-4

Review. The abnormal Q wave in Figure 16-3 has a duration of 0.03 sec in lead I. Figure 16-5 shows this complex together with related anterolateral leads aVL and V_6, both with Q waves due to old myocardial infarction. The serial complexes in Figure 16-4 show progressive development of a large Q wave in a patient with inferior infarction.

Myocardial infarction of the ventricular septum or posterior left ventricular wall typically causes abnormal initial QRS forces in the horizontal plane, usually most evident in leads V_1 and V_2. Figure 16-6(A) illustrates the effect of septal or anteroseptal infarction. When normal initial septal depolarization does not occur, the first QRS forces are directed posteriorly as diagramed in a horizontal cross-section of

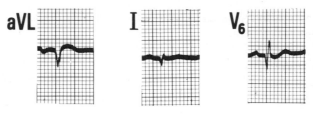

Figure 16-5

the ventricle viewed from above. Septal infarction, therefore, changes the normal RS complex in V_1 to a QS configuration. QS complexes may be confined to leads V_1 and V_2 or may extend to leads V_3 and V_4, generally reflecting the size of the infarcted zone. Within weeks or months after the event, small R waves may reappear in these leads, resulting in a chronic pattern of delayed R wave progression as the only residual evidence of an old anteroseptal or anterior infarct.

Figure 16-6(B) shows the effects of posterior wall infarction. When normal posterior wall forces are eliminated, unopposed septal forces, directed anteriorly, result in a tall and abnormally wide R wave in leads V_1 and V_2.

For an uncomplicated first infarction, the EKG identifies the involved LV zone with reasonable accuracy. Exceptions are that small

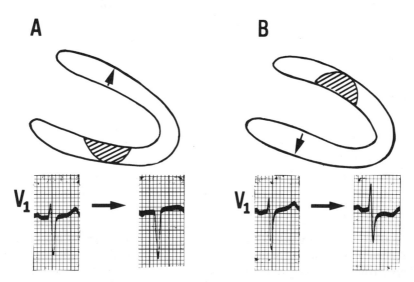

Figure 16-6 QRS effects of (A) anteroseptal and (B) posterior wall myocardial infarction, with diagram of LV in transverse cross-section viewed from above.

infarcts or silent zone infarcts in anatomic sites not closely related to EKG lead positions may cause no well-defined EKG abnormalities. EKG findings are less reliable in distinguishing transmural infarcts that involve the full ventricular wall thickness from intramural infarcts. In general, infarctions that cause typical QRS abnormalities are relatively large and transmural. Intramural or subendocardial infarction may cause well-defined ST segment and T wave abnormalities without alteration of the QRS complex. Right ventricular infarcts may accompany extensive LV infarction, but cannot be diagnosed reliably by a routine 12-lead EKG.

The following lists summarize frequent or important causes of two common QRS abnormalities:

1. *Tall R waves in lead V₁:*
   a. Counterclockwise rotation, no heart disease.
   b. Posterior wall infarction.
   c. RV conduction delay.
   d. RVH.
   e. WPW syndrome with anteriorly directed delta wave.
2. *Delayed precordial R wave progression:*
   a. Clockwise rotation, no heart disease.
   b. Old anteroseptal infarction.
   c. LV conduction delay.
   d. LVH.

Complete the following sentences:

1. _____ BBB does not alter initial QRS forces and, therefore, does not influence the accuracy of _____ wave criteria for myocardial infarction.

2. Posterior wall infarction results in unopposed initial QRS forces directed _____ and displayed as a tall _____ wave in lead _____ .

3. WPW syndrome may mimic the QRS pattern of inferior infarction when the _____ wave results from an abnormal LV depolarization force that is directed _____ .

Review. Q wave criteria for infarction are valid in the presence of RBBB, which does not alter initial QRS forces. LBBB invalidates Q wave criteria. A tall R wave in V₁ may result from posterior wall infarction. When delta wave forces are directed superiorly, they are represented by a Q wave in inferior leads and may mimic inferior wall infarction.

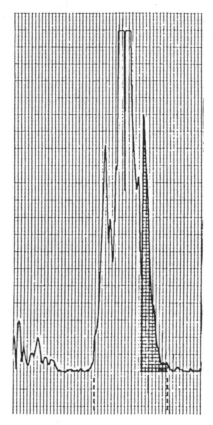

Figure 16-7 Normal signal-averaged QRS complex.

Another QRS abnormality related to myocardial infarction is the presence of late high frequency, low amplitude (HFLA) QRS components. These waves result from slow spread of depolarization in small areas of myocardium adjacent to or within the infarct zone. Because slow, asynchronous conduction is a setting for reentry, the presence of HFLA potentials correlates with the risk of postinfarction ventricular tachycardia and fibrillation.

Computerized processing of the QRS complex at high recording speed is required to demonstrate HFLA potentials. To minimize electrical interference from extraneous sources, the computer program analyzes a large number of complexes and develops a composite complex recorded at 200 mm/sec. The computer also measures the duration and amplitude of QRS forces, expressing amplitude of the late forces (terminal 40 msec of the QRS complex) as a mathematically derived variable, the root mean square (RMS). Current normal standards for the signal-averaged QRS complex include total duration less than 114 msec, dura-

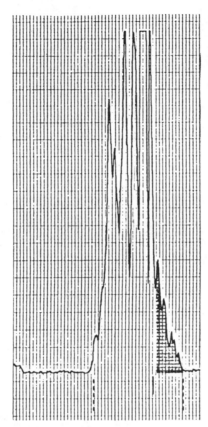

Figure 16-8 Signal-averaged QRS complex in a patient with paroxysmal ventricular tachycardia showing abnormal late HFLA potentials (shaded area).

tion of HFLA potentials less than 39 msec, and RMS amplitude of the terminal 40 msec less than 20 μV.

Examine Figure 16-7, the display of a normal signal-averaged QRS complex calibrated at 1 cm = 0.01 mV. The complex is wide because the recording speed is 200 msec. The terminal 40 msec of the complex is shaded. The RMS voltage for this segment is 34 μV. The duration of low amplitude signals less than 40 μV is 28 msec.

Figure 16-8 shows a signal-averaged QRS complex of a patient with ventricular tachycardia. The RMS voltage of the terminal 40 msec is abnormally low at 15 μV, and the HFLA duration is prolonged at 45 msec.

4 | Abnormal ST Segments

Lesson 17

ST Segment Elevation

ST segment elevation is a cardinal EKG abnormality that is often difficult to interpret. In one form, it is a common innocuous finding in healthy young people. In other instances, ST elevation is a hallmark of CAD, of pericarditis, or of ventricular aneurysm.

ST elevation in a normal young person, referred to as repolarization variant or *early repolarization,* occurs principally in leads with high QRS voltage and is usually most prominent in lead V_5 or V_6. Typically, the elevated segment has a smoothly rounded downward convexity as shown in Figure 17-1. The degree of elevation measured from the level of the PR segment is usually slight, but may exceed 4 mm. The J point is also elevated but indistinct because of the smooth transition between R wave and ST segment. Normal variant ST elevation may be an unstable finding, varying in degree and at times clearing completely on repeated EKGs of the same patient. Its greatest importance lies in the risk of mistaking normal variation for a pathologic abnormality.

In contrast, ST elevation that results from myocardial ischemia or infarction commonly has serious implications. When ST elevation in this category is transient and subsides in 15 min or less, it often correlates with a period of reversible coronary artery obstruction due to

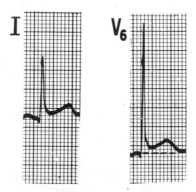

Figure 17-1 Normal variant ST segment elevation (early repolarization).

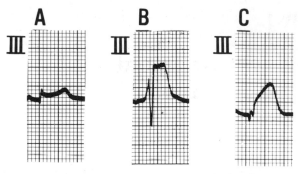

Figure 17-2   ST elevation due to acute myocardial ischemia or infarction.

arteriospasm, as seen in Prinzmetal's angina. When ST segment elevation develops and persists in a patient with anginal pain, it is a manifestation of acute myocardial infarction.

Figure 17-2 illustrates different ST segment configurations associated with acute myocardial ischemia or infarction. The elevated ST
segment in Figure 17-2(A) is slightly curved and shows distinct J point
elevation, an appearance commonly seen in the early hours after onset

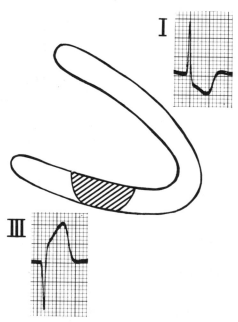

Figure 17-3   Reciprocal ST abnormalities due to acute inferior myocardial
infarction with diagramatic anterior view of the LV in frontal
cross-section.

of myocardial infarction. Figure 17-2(B) shows an extensive flat, or horizontal, ST elevation due to coronary arteriospasm. In this patient, who later had normal coronary arteriograms, the marked EKG abnormality subsided within 2 min and was not associated with chest pain or other symptoms. In Figure 17-2(C), the ST segment shows upsloping elevation. The T wave is tall and the junction of the ST segment and T wave is not distinct. This configuration also may be seen in the early phase of acute infarction.

An important associated abnormality that aids in assessment of ST elevation due to myocardial ischemia is the frequent presence of reciprocal ST depression. In Lesson 4, you learned the principle of reciprocal EKG waves. Localized LV injury often results in oppositely directed waves in lead groups that have opposite anatomic positions. Figure 17-3 illustrates this relationship for ST abnormalities during inferior myocardial infarction. ST elevation in inferior leads and ST depression in the anterolateral leads are reciprocal, or mutual, manifestations of the same electrical force. Reciprocal waves are commonly a feature of myocardial infarction because the infarction is typically localized to one region of the LV. Reciprocal changes are unlikely to result from a diffuse pathologic process that involves the ventricle uniformly or at a number of different sites.

Complete the following sentences:

1. In Figure 17-4, the lead III complex indicated by letter _____ suggests the need for prompt hospitalization, especially if the patient has chest pain and if the EKG shows _____ ST depression in leads I and aVL.

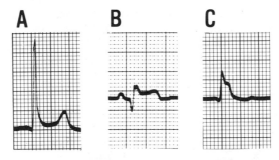

Figure 17-4

2. Figure 17-5 shows QRS duration of _____ sec and an R wave configuration in lead I typical of _____ . Lead V_1 shows a wide notched QS wave and an _____ ST segment.

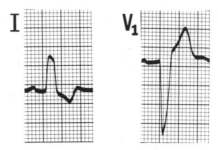

Figure 17-5

Review. The complex in Figure 17-4(B) shows ST elevation in lead III that strongly suggests inferior wall ischemia or infarction, especially if reciprocal ST depression is present in anterolateral leads I and aVL. Figure 17-5 shows LBBB with QRS duration 0.14 sec. The upsloping ST elevation in lead V_1 is secondary to the conduction abnormality.

Another important cause of ST elevation is acute pericarditis. In patients with acute chest pain, diagnostic confusion results at times because the ST elevation of ischemia or infarction and that of acute pericarditis may be similar. In pericarditis, ST elevation is present in several lead groups and is not accompanied by reciprocal ST depression. Figure 17-6 illustrates the diffuse ST elevation of acute pericarditis. As inflammation subsides, the ST segment returns to the baseline.

When an extensive myocardial infarction leads to a large scar or left ventricular aneurysm, ST elevation may persist indefinitely in EKG leads related to the involved LV segment. These leads also display Q or QS waves due to the infarct. Figure 17-7 illustrates ST abnormalities associated with an anterior LV aneurysm. A distinguishing feature of this pattern is its stability, with little change in ST configuration over a period of months or years.

A minor degree of ST elevation may occur, especially in the right precordial leads, for a variety of less well-defined reasons. Figure

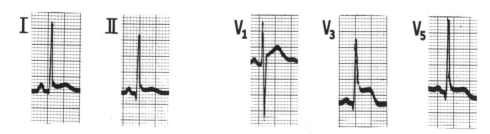

Figure 17-6   ST elevation due to acute pericarditis.

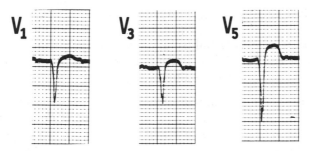

Figure 17-7 ST elevation due to LV aneurysm.

17-8(A) illustrates innocuous ST elevation in V_1 associated with an r′ wave that elevates the J point. Figure 17-8(B) shows primary ST depression in V_6 and reciprocal ST elevation in V_1 in a patient with high QRS voltage due to LVH.

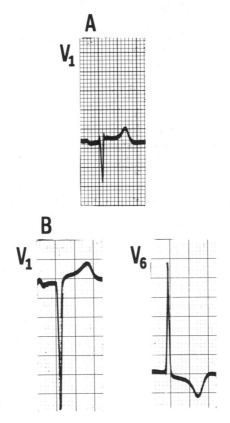

Figure 17-8 ST segment elevation in lead V_1 (A) with rSr′ QRS complex and (B) as reciprocal abnormality related to ST segment depression in V_6.

Complete the following sentences:

1. In addition to myocardial ischemia or injury, important pathologic causes of ST elevation are _____ _____ and ventricular _____ .

2. Figure 17-9 shows complexes from an emergency room EKG of a 32-year-old man complaining of chest pain that developed after a hard football tackle. Traumatic pericarditis was considered, but excluded because _____ ST depression is present in lead I.

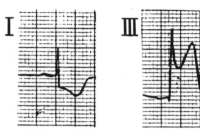

Figure 17-9

Review.   Acute pericarditis and left ventricular aneurysm cause ST elevation. Reciprocal ST depression in lead I of Figure 17-9 confirms the EKG diagnosis of acute inferior myocardial infarction that occurred 2 hours before this patient reached the emergency room.

Lesson 18

ST Segment Depression Due to Subendocardial Ischemia / Stress Test Interpretation

As in the case of ST elevation, interpretation of ST displacement below the EKG baseline commonly depends on the clinical setting, as well as degree of displacement, ST configuration, stability of the abnormality, and association with other EKG findings. CAD is the most important cause of ST depression. When elicited by exercise, the degree of ST depression in CAD patients correlates with the extent of myocardial ischemia, particularly in the subendocardial zone of the left ventricle. Subendocardial fibers are especially vulnerable to imbalances of myocardial oxygen supply and demand.

Figure 18-1 illustrates three varieties of ST depression, each with depression of the J point. In Figure 18-1(A), the depressed ST segment is flat or horizontal. The degree of depression is 4.5 mm measured from the top of the ST segment to the top of an EKG baseline extended from the PR segment. The degree of upsloping ST depression, Figure 18-1(B), is 1.0 mm measured at a point 0.08 sec after the J point. For downsloping ST depression, Figure 18-1(C), measure the degree of J point depres-

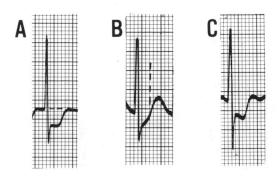

Figure 18-1 Configuration of depressed ST segments: (A) horizontal, (B) upsloping with J point depression, and (C) downsloping.

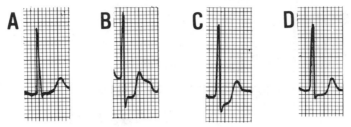

Figure 18-2 ST abnormalities during exercise; (A) before exercise, (B) at peak stress, (C) 3 min after exercise, and (D) 8 min after exercise.

sion, 4.0 mm. ST depression provoked by exercise is usually most prominent in leads with tall R waves. Anatomic correlations between the abnormal lead group and the ischemic LV segment are generally unreliable.

Figure 18-2 illustrates a typical sequence of ST depression and gradual recovery after exercise. At peak stress [Figure 18-2(B)], 5.0-mm horizontal ST depression is present. During recovery, ST depression commonly becomes upsloping or downsloping. In this example, 1.5-mm horizontal ST depression is still present 8 min after exercise [Figure 18-2(D)].

Statistically derived criteria for abnormal ST depression during exercise should be viewed broadly. As in the case of many EKG findings, ST changes during stress form a spectrum that is not readily divided by a single criterion into normal and abnormal groups. ST depression of 1.0-mm at a high level of stress does not reliably indicate the presence of CAD in an asymptomatic patient. Horizontal or downsloping ST depression of 2.0 mm or more during mild to moderate stress correlates with major CAD in the absence of other explanation. ST depression during exercise cannot be reliably interpreted if the patient is taking digitalis or when a pretest EKG shows major abnormalities, especially LBBB.

Complete the following sentences:

1. ST depression in Figure 18-3 is _____ mm
   and _____ in configuration at heart rate _____ bpm.
   It is probable that this patient's coronary arteriograms will
   show _____ .

Review. Figure 18-3 shows 3.5-mm downsloping ST depression measured from the PR segment to the J point at a heart rate of 105 bpm. This abnormality at a low level of stress correlates with major CAD.

An exercise stress test is a clinical experiment of great value when properly conducted in appropriately selected patients. For each patient,

---

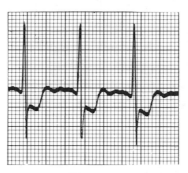

Figure 18-3

the purpose of the test must be clearly formulated. Important variables include not only the degree of ST segment depression and its configuration, but also the level of myocardial oxygen demand as reflected in maximal heart rate achieved, or in the double product of peak heart rate × peak systolic blood pressure. Other observations to be routinely reported include duration and degree of exercise, symptoms during the test, time of onset and total duration of ST abnormality, and blood pressure response to exercise. Maximal heart rate achieved is commonly reported as a percentage of statistically predicted maximal rate for patient age.

Confusion may follow when stress test results are reported as "positive," "negative," or "inconclusive because of inadequate stress." Positive or negative reports imply the presence or absence of CAD. In fact, an abnormal stress response may reflect a variety of other cardiac disorders, or may occur in the absence of detectable heart disease. Definition of adequate stress should reflect the purpose of the test. When an exercise test is used to estimate the likelihood of CAD in an asymptomatic patient, adequate stress is often equated to an achieved heart rate equal to 85% of age-predicted maximal rate.

Lesson 19

Other Causes of ST Segment Depression

Downward displacement of the ST segment is a common abnormality with a wide range of possible causes. It may be an isolated finding on an otherwise normal EKG, but associated T wave abnormalities are often present. ST depression regularly occurs as a secondary effect of LBBB or as a manifestation of ventricular hypertrophy. It may also result from myocardial inflammation, electrolyte disorders, or drug effects. When the abnormality has no distinct explanation, it is classed as *nonspecific*.

Figure 19-1(A) shows typical ST abnormalities in a patient with LBBB. Note the prominent downsloping ST depression that accompanies the wide QRS complex in a lead with tall R wave. This ST depression is secondary to an abnormal ventricular depolarization sequence and improves when the QRS complex narrows [Figure 19-1(B)]. Figure 19-2 illustrates secondary ST abnormalities in a patient with WPW syndrome.

In Figure 19-3, LVH is the cause of ST depression, again seen principally in a lead with tall R wave, which in this example has amplitude of 54 mm. This manifestation of LVH, sometimes referred to as *LV strain pattern,* tends to occur most prominently in patients with ventricular pressure overload. For an individual patient on different occasions, the degree of ST depression may correlate with the degree of overload present. Figure 19-4 illustrates improvement of an ST abnor-

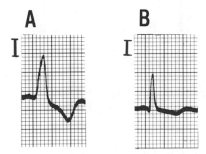

Figure 19-1   ST segment depression secondary to LBBB (A).

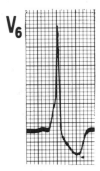

Figure 19-2 ST depression secondary to WPW syndrome.

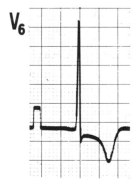

Figure 19-3 ST segment depression secondary to LVH. Note that the calibration artifact indicates half standard calibration, 1 mV = 0.5 mm. The standard R wave amplitude is therefore twice the measured amplitude.

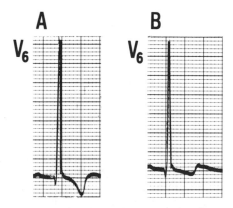

Figure 19-4 (A) ST depression in hypertensive heart disease with (B) improvement after antihypertensive therapy.

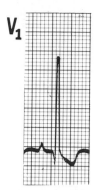

Figure 19-5 ST depression secondary to RVH.

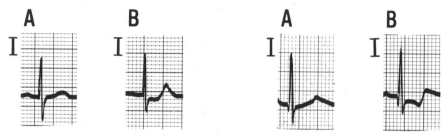

Figure 19-6 ST configuration (A) before and (B) after digitalis therapy.

mality after successful treatment of a hypertensive patient. In Figure 19-5, lead V_1 shows a large R wave due to RVH accompanied by ST depression, or RV strain pattern.

ST depression is the principal change in the ventricular EKG complex that is associated with digitalis therapy, which also tends to shorten the QT interval. This finding, termed *digitalis effect,* does not correlate well with therapeutic response or with serum drug level of the digitalis glycoside. Figure 19-6 shows two configurations of the depressed ST segment that are typical of digitalis effect.

Complete the following sentences:

1. In Figure 19-7, the QRS complex in lead V_1 shows _____ . The ST segment is _____ .

2. In Figure 19-8, the apparent ST depression is caused by superimposed waves of _____ .

3. In lead I of Figure 19-9 _____ ST depression reflects the ST elevation in the inferior leads during acute inferior myocardial infarction.

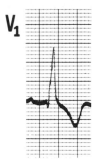

Figure 19-7

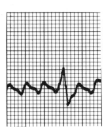

Figure 19-8

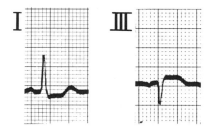

Figure 19-9

Review. Figure 19-7 illustrates RBBB associated with a downsloping ST segment. The atrial flutter waves in Figure 19-8 cause an apparent ST depression. Figure 19-9 shows reciprocal lead I ST depression in a patient with inferior infarction.

5 | Abnormal T Waves

Lesson 20

Nonspecific T Wave Abnormalities

Many pathologic and physiologic events may alter ventricular repolarization and cause T wave abnormalities. Abnormal T wave inversion or flattening is described as *nonspecific* when the range of possible etiologies is broad and available evidence does not permit more precise interpretation. This term may be deceptive. "Nonspecific T wave abnormality" may be a subtle manifestation of coronary artery disease. In other clinical settings, the term may describe an innocuous finding that should not be regarded as evidence of heart disease.

In Lesson 8, you learned that T wave inversion is generally abnormal when present in a lead that displays an upright QRS complex. Interpretation of abnormally inverted T waves depends on other findings, such as:

Depth of T wave inversion

T wave configuration

Number of leads and lead group involved

Coexisting QRS or ST abnormalities

Details of the clinical setting

Examine Figure 20-1, the routine EKG of an asymptomatic normotensive 45-year-old man. Complexes are arranged according to lead axes in the frontal plane [Figure 20-1(A)] and horizontal plane [Figure 20-1(B)]. First evaluate the QRS complex, which shows normal width and configuration, with a frontal plane axis of 0°. Slight T wave inversion is present in lead a VL, which shows a tall R wave. In the chest leads, note that the T wave in lead V_1 is taller than the T wave in lead V_6. This tracing shows a relatively common form of anterolateral T wave abnormality. The T wave direction, or axis, diverges from the QRS axis in both the limb leads and the chest leads. Unless clinical findings clarify the cause of this abnormality, the pattern is considered nonspecific, for it may occur in many forms of heart disease and also in persons who have no detectable cardiovascular disorder.

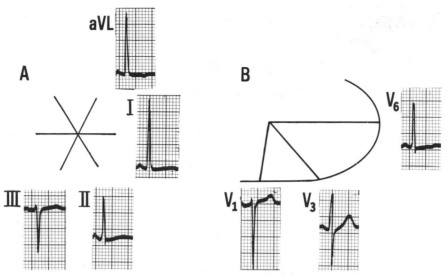

Figure 20-1 Nonspecific anterolateral T wave abnormality in (A) frontal plane leads and (B) horizontal plane leads.

Complete the following sentences:

1. When the T wave axis and _____ _____ are divergent, the T wave becomes flat or _____ in leads that display tall _____ waves.

2. When the T wave axis is −60°, T wave inversion will be present in the _____ lead group.

3. In the horizontal plane, the T wave in lead _____ will be taller than the T wave in lead _____ when the T wave axis has an abnormal anterior direction.

Review. In evaluating T wave inversion or flattening in either the limb leads or chest leads, it is important to note the relation of T wave direction to QRS direction. When these waves diverge abnormally,

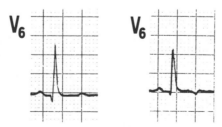

Figure 20-2 Nonspecific T wave inversion in a healthy subject; (A) upright T wave in supine position; (B) inverted T waves on standing.

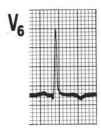

Figure 20-3 Nonspecific T wave inversion with symmetric contour.

leads with prominent R waves will show flat or inverted T waves. An upward deviation of T wave axis to −60° results in inferior lead T wave inversion.

Two categories of T wave inversion may be broadly defined on the basis of configuration and depth of inversion. In the first category are mild to moderate abnormalities reflecting autonomic or metabolic responses to a variety of nonpathologic stimuli, such as change of position, hyperventilation, or the postprandial state. T wave configuration is typically asymmetric, often with slight ST segment depression. These changes are transient and resolve soon after the stimulus terminates. Figure 20-2 illustrates nonspecific T wave abnormality due to change of position in a healthy person.

In the second category of nonspecific T wave inversion, the abnormality is more pronounced and symmetric, as illustrated in Figure 20-3. This finding usually has a pathologic basis, but may result from a wide variety of diseases, including extracardiac conditions such as acute biliary tract disease. The abnormality is commonly confined to a single lead group and may be temporary or chronic.

Complete the following sentences:

1. Figure 20-4 shows chest lead complexes of a 20-year-old man recorded several hours after emergency treatment for a chest stab wound. Abnormal T wave inversion is present in leads _____ . Although this T wave abnormality is _____ , it is consistent with cardiac trauma in this clinical setting.

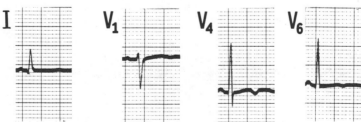

Figure 20-4

2. Figure 20-5 shows complexes recorded during treatment of a 24-year-old woman who was resuscitated after an overdose of sedative drugs. The QRS complex is _____ . Nonspecific T wave inversion is present in leads _____ , _____ , and _____ .

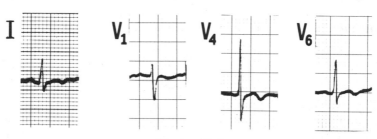

Figure 20-5

Review. In Figure 20-4, T wave inversion is present in leads V_4 and V_6 and the T wave in lead I is flat. Although these findings are nonspecific, they may be a clue to cardiac trauma in a patient with a penetrating chest wound. The QRS complex is normal in Figure 20-5, and nonspecific T wave inversion is present in leads I, V_4, and V_6. The slight T wave inversion in lead V_1 is not an abnormality.

POSTEXTRASYSTOLIC T WAVE INVERSION

Figure 20-6 illustrates a T wave abnormality that may occur after a premature beat. The first two complexes are normal. Complex X, a ventricular extrasystole, displays a wide QRS due to ectopic origin of

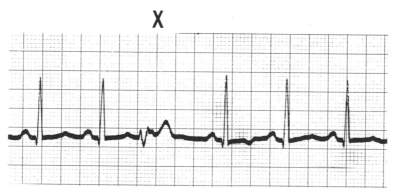

Figure 20-6   Postextrasystolic T wave inversion.

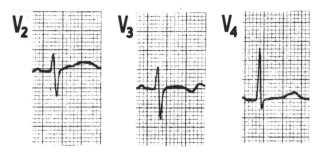

Figure 20-7   Isolated T wave inversion, V₃.

depolarization. The following complex is a normal sinus beat with postextrasystolic T wave inversion that is present for only one cardiac cycle. After a prolonged tachyarrhythmia, nonspecific T wave inversion occasionally persists for minutes or hours after sinus rhythm returns, a finding sometimes termed the *posttachycardia syndrome*.

ISOLATED T WAVE INVERSION

Figure 20-7 illustrates an uncommon phenomenon that may occur in the absence of heart disease. The T wave in lead V_3 is inverted, although in adjacent leads V_2 and V_4 the T wave is upright. The cause of isolated T wave inversion is not well defined.

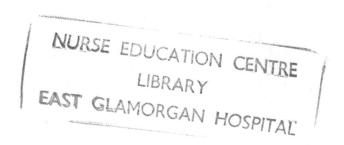

Lesson 21

T Wave Abnormalities Due to Coronary Artery Disease

The natural history of atherosclerotic CAD varies widely. The complex spectrum of this disease ranges from clinical latency, when symptoms or other manifestations are absent in spite of major coronary stenosis or occlusion, to the dramatic acute syndrome of myocardial infarction. EKG manifestations of CAD are equally varied and at times diverge from other clinical findings. A routine EKG of an symptomatic patient may reveal abnormalities due to CAD. Conversely, the EKG may show little or no abnormality during a major acute coronary event.

CAD commonly causes repolarization abnormalities. In the past, T wave inversion has been considered an indication of myocardial ischemia, but this correlation is not reliable. As usually defined in CAD, ischemia is an oxygenation imbalance that occurs when cellular metabolic demands exceed oxygen supply because of inadequate regional coronary flow. Unless this condition progresses to infarction, it is typically transient and reversible. The principal EKG effect of ischemia is an ST segment shift above or below the baseline. T wave abnormalities relate to more diverse effects of CAD on the LV myocardium. Stable T wave inversion, for example, may result from an old myocardial infarction rather than reversible ischemia.

In this area of electrocardiography, it is important to emphasize the objective and subjective aspects of interpretation. An initial objective step involves identification of abnormal T wave inversion, its depth and contour and comparison with the patient's previous EKGs, if available, to discover whether the abnormality is new or progressive. At times a T wave inversion pattern can be considered strong direct evidence that CAD is present. More commonly the meaning of a T wave abnormality depends on details of the clinical setting, especially the characteristics of chest pain, if present. The interpreter must use all available facts to estimate the likelihood that an observed T wave abnormality is in fact a manifestation of CAD and to assess its physiologic basis. In this judgmental aspect of interpretation, there is room for well-considered differences of opinion among different electrocardiographers interpreting the same EKG.

Complete the following questions:

1. In Figure 21-1, the shape of the deeply inverted T wave is _____ .

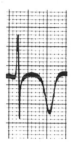

Figure 21-1

2. Figure 21-2 shows T wave inversion in leads _____ through _____ , in which QRS complexes have a _____ direction. The transition zone for this series of precordial leads is between leads _____ and _____ . The shape of the inverted T waves is _____ . In a 24-year-old woman, these findings suggest a nonpathologic persistent _____ pattern.

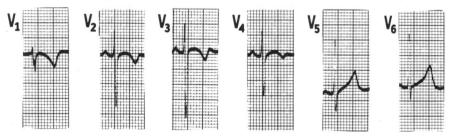

Figure 21-2

Review. T wave inversion in Figure 21-1 is symmetric and strongly supports a diagnosis of acute CAD in a patient with chest pain, although other diseases may occasionally cause this abnormality. Leads V_1 through V_4 of Figure 21-2 show asymmetric T wave inversion in leads with negative QRS complexes, consistent with a persistent juvenile pattern. Transition zone lies between leads V_4 and V_5.

Two categories of T wave abnormality due to CAD are:

1. T wave inversion in the absence of QRS abnormalities. T wave contour is typically symmetric, as Figure 21-3(A) illustrates. When the ST segment is slightly elevated, the inverted T wave turns sharply downward at the ST-T junction as in Figure 21-3(B). The degree of inversion may be minimal or pronounced. The abnormality often involves a single anatomic lead group and may be stable or unstable. On serial tracings, the T wave inversion often progresses or regresses over a period of days or weeks.

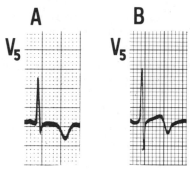

Figure 21-3   T wave inversion due to CAD.

2. T wave abnormalities that accompany QRS and ST abnormalities of myocardial infarction. During typical acute transmural infarction, sequential Q wave and ST segment changes are accompanied by the following T wave abnormalities:
   a. Immediate, or "hyperacute," stage (minutes to hours after coronary occlusion): tall T waves, with upsloping ST elevation.
   b. Acute stage (hours to days): progressive T wave inversion.
   c. Late stage (weeks to months): T wave inversion regresses and may resolve completely.

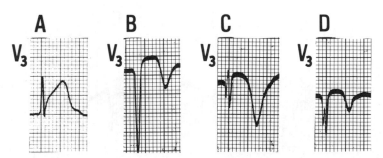

Figure 21-4   Evolution of anterior myocardial infarction: (A) immediate stage, (B) second day, (C) third day, and (D) fourteenth day.

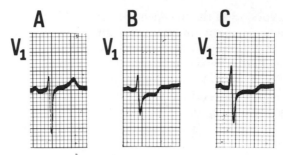

Figure 21-5 Evolution of posterior myocardial infarction: (A) before infarction, (B) first day, and (C) fifth day.

Identify this sequence of T wave changes in Figure 21-4, which illustrates typical evolution of transmural anterior myocardial infarction.

Recall that infarction of the posterior LV wall causes abnormalities in anterior leads that are opposite in direction to those observed during anterior infarction. In lead V_1, posterior infarcts result in a prominent R wave, rather than a Q wave. Similarly, ST and T wave abnormalities of posterior infarction are opposite to those of anterior infarction. As Figure 21-5 illustrates, acute posterior wall infarcts cause ST depression in anterior leads. T waves are inverted or flat during the acute stage and become upright as the infarct pattern evolves.

Complete the following sentences:

1. In Figure 21-6(A), the lead III ST-T wave abnormality indicates the _____ stage of _____ wall left ventricular infarction.

2. The ST-T wave abnormalities in Figures 21-6(B) and 21-6(C) occur during the _____ stage of infarction, at a time interval of hours or _____ after the onset of symptoms.

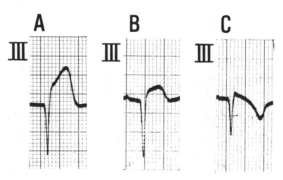

Figure 21-6

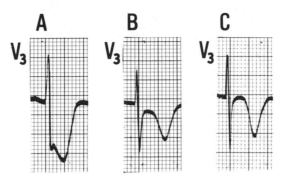

Figure 21-7 Evolution of acute anterior non–Q wave myocardial infarction: (A) first day, (B) second day, and (C) third day.

Review. The upsloping ST elevation and tall T wave in Figure 21-6(A) are consistent with the immediate or hyperacute stage of inferior infarction. The presence of a deep QS wave at this stage is atypical. Figures 21-6(B) and 21-6(C) illustrate acute stage evolution and were recorded on the second and third days after onset of symptoms.

Another pattern of sequential ST and T wave abnormalities may appear without Q waves during the course of intramural infarction. This "T wave infarction" pattern may also be an atypical manifestation of transmural infarction. Although the pattern of evolution is variable, typical findings include:

Immediate stage—marked horizontal ST depression

Acute stage—progressive symmetric T wave inversion; ST segment returns toward baseline

Late stage—T wave inversion regresses and may resolve

Figure 21-7 illustrates typical evolution of acute anterior non–Q wave infarction.

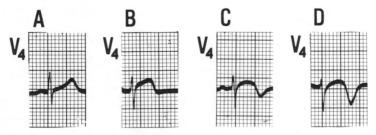

Figure 21-8 Evolution of anterior subepicardial myocardial infarction: (A) before infarction, (B) first day, (C) third day, and (D) fifth day.

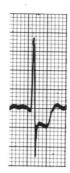

Figure 21-9

Figure 21-8 illustrates a less common non–Q wave infarction pattern in which ST elevation precedes progressive T wave inversion. This finding may correlate with subepicardial location of the infarct. Note that R wave amplitude decreases, but Q waves do not appear.

Complete the following sentences:

1. During acute non–Q wave infarction involving subendocardial fibers, ST _____ occurs initially. Subepicardial infarcts cause ST _____ .

2. Figure 21-9 shows downsloping ST depression of _____ mm. This finding may reflect transient subendocardial _____ . ST depression persists when _____ has occurred, with progressive T wave _____ on serial tracings.

Review. Subendocardial ischemia or injury correlates with ST depression. ST elevation accompanies subepicardial injury. ST depression in Figure 21-9 is 3.5 mm and may reflect either transient ischemia, or if persistent, non-Q wave infarction, with progressive T wave inversion to be expected as the infarct evolves.

Lesson 22

Other Well-Defined T Wave Abnormalities

Interpretation of abnormal T wave inversion or flattening is among the most frequent and difficult problems of electrocardiography. As discussed in Lessons 20 and 21, these abnormalities may be nonspecific when the range of possible causes is wide, or their contour and clinical context may suggest CAD. Lesson 22 concerns abnormal T wave patterns that are consistent with other well-defined causes including ventricular hypertrophy, BBB, pericarditis, and intracranial hemorrhage.

ST and T wave abnormalities are an important manifestation of LVH or RVH. They are most pronounced in leads with tall R waves. As Figure 22-1 illustrates, the severity and contour of these abnormalities are variable. In general, the degree of abnormality correlates with the severity of hypertrophy or of ventricular pressure overload. Major degrees of downsloping ST depression and T wave inversion have adverse clinical implications, as suggested by the term *ventricular strain* sometimes used to describe this pattern. As you learned in Lesson 15, the primary EKG manifestations of ventricular hypertrophy involve the QRS complex. In an appropriate clinical setting, ST-T wave abnormalities may at times be attributed to this cause when the tracing shows no QRS evidence of hypertrophy.

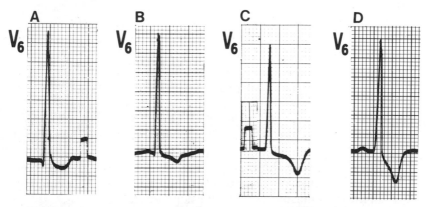

Figure 22-1 ST-T wave abnormalities due to LVH in four patients.

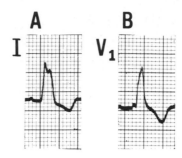

Figure 22-2 ST-T wave abnormalities secondary to (A) LBBB and (B) RBBB.

In Lesson 13, you learned about QRS deformities due to BBB. This major depolarization abnormality is regularly accompanied by repolarization abnormalities, as illustrated in Figure 22-2. ST depression and T wave inversion are again most prominent in leads with tall R waves. The degree of abnormality is of little importance. These changes are a secondary result of BBB and do not require further interpretation. They often obscure primary ST-T wave abnormalities due to CAD or other causes.

Complete the following sentences:

1. In Figure 22-3, the large R wave in lead V_1 is _____ sec in duration. In this young patient with congenital heart disease, the deep T wave inversion results from _____ _____ hypertrophy.

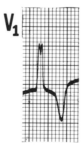

Figure 22-3

2. The QRS complex in Figure 22-4 is _____ sec in duration. The short PR interval confirms that the ST-T wave abnormality accompanies abnormal ventricular depolarization in the _____ _____ _____ syndrome.

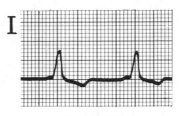

Figure 22-4

Review. The R wave duration is 0.09 sec in Figure 22-3, which shows RVH and strain. In Figure 22-4, the QRS is 0.12 sec wide because of WPW syndrome.

Pericarditis is another cause of T wave inversion. In Lesson 17, you learned that ST elevation is the cardinal EKG manifestation of acute pericardial inflammation. As inflammation subsides, the ST segment returns to the baseline. Typically, T wave inversion follows, as illustrated in Figure 22-5. T wave inversion may persist indefinitely in chronic pericarditis.

An unusual degree of T wave inversion may occur in patients with acute subarachnoid hemorrhage, as illustrated in Figure 22-6. The T

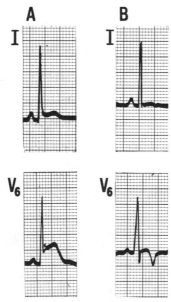

Figure 22-5 ST-T wave abnormalities due to acute pericarditis: (A) first day; (B) fourth day.

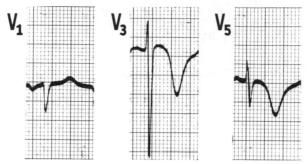

Figure 22-6 T wave inversion in a 29-year-old patient with subarachnoid hemorrhage.

waves are wide and symmetric. This finding is related to sympathetic nervous system effects on ventricular repolarization. Similar abnormalities may accompany surgical manipulation of cervical sympathetic ganglia. Note the similarity of this pattern to the deep, symmetric T wave inversion due to coronary disease illustrated in Figure 21-7.

6 | Abnormal Impulse Formation and Conduction Disorders

Lesson 23

Dysfunction of Automatic Pacing Tissues

The SA node, AV junction, and ventricular Purkinje fibers normally share the property of spontaneous impulse formation at varying inherent rates. These pacing tissues differ somewhat in their physiologic responses and in the pathologic conditions that lead to their dysfunction. The rate of SA node impulse formation is highly sensitive to variation in autonomic nerve activity, especially through cardiac branches of the vagus nerve. Vagal stimulation slows both the SA and AV junctional pacemakers. Thyroid hormone and circulating catecholamines stimulate automatic fibers. Fibrosis and other forms of degeneration may involve all structures of the pacing and conduction system, a common finding in elderly patients. Pacing tissue dysfunction is rarely catastrophic unless advanced heart disease is present. Inappropriate acceleration or slowing of an intrinsic pacemaker, however, may give evidence of an underlying cardiac or extracardiac disorder or of an adverse drug effect.

SA BLOCK

Slow sinus rhythm occasionally results from SA exit block. In this form of SA node dysfunction, impulse formation within the node is not primarily impaired, but some of the impulses formed are not conducted out of the node to the atria. The EKG shows sinus rhythm that may be irregular because of changing conduction ratios through the perinodal fibers (PNF). In Figure 23-1, the ladder diagram illustrates intermittent 2:1 SA exit block. Spontaneous depolarization within the node is regular. The third and fifth impulses are blocked and do not activate the atria. No P waves appear. The long P-to-P intervals are exactly twice the length of the short P-to-P intervals.

To interpret cardiac rhythm systematically, first identify P waves and note their timing in relation to each other. Then note the timing and configuration of QRS complexes. A narrow QRS ($\leq$0.10 sec) indicates supraventricular origin of depolarization. An abnormally wide

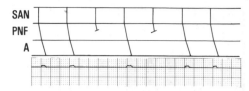

Figure 23-1   Intermittent 2 : 1 SA exit block.

complex may indicate BBB or ventricular ectopic origin of depolarization. Then measure the PRI and note any variation in the relationship
between P waves and QRS complexes that follow them.

Complete the following sentences:

1. In Figure 23-2, the first P-to-P interval is _____ sec. The
   second P-to-P interval is _____ sec. The ratio of the long
   interval to the short interval suggests SA exit block
   with _____ to _____ conduction. The QRS duration
   of _____ sec indicates that depolarization enters the
   ventricles through the _____ bundle and that conduction
   through the bundle branches is normal. The PRI is _____
   and the AV conduction ratio is _____ to _____ .

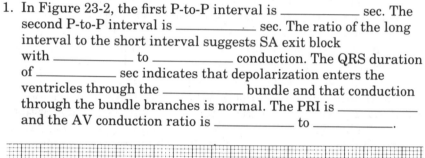

Figure 23-2

2. Slow SA rhythm usually results from depressed _____
   impulse formation, but may also reflect SA _____ .

3. In Figure 23-3, _____ waves are absent. The QRS
   duration is _____ sec. The ventricular complexes are
   totally _____ in timing. This supraventricular arrhythmia
   is _____ _____ .

Review.   In Figure 23-2, the long P-to-P interval of 1.84 sec is approximately twice the short interval of 0.88 sec, suggesting a 2 : 1 SA exit
block. The QRS duration is 0.10 sec, indicating rapid ventricular depo-

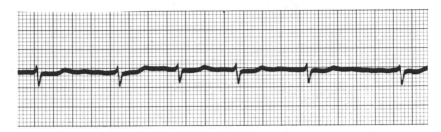

Figure 23-3

larization from the His bundle and its branches. The PRI is constant, 0.14 sec, and AV conduction is 1 : 1. Depressed automatic impulse formation is the usual cause of slow sinus rhythms, which may also result from SA exit block. In Figure 23-3, the absence of P waves and the totally irregular QRS complexes of supraventricular origin, 0.08 sec in duration, identify AF.

ACTIVITY OF SECONDARY PACEMAKERS

Automatic pacing tissues in the AV junction can control heart rhythm under two general circumstances. In one circumstance, the junctional pacemaker has a passive role. It forms impulses at its normal inherent rate. It controls heart rhythm either because the SA node has slowed to a lesser rate or because SA node impulses encounter a conduction block and do not reach the secondary pacemaker. In a second circumstance, the junctional pacemaker controls heart rhythm because it actively accelerates to an abnormal rate that exceeds the normal rate of the SA node.

Figure 23-4 illustrates two patterns of AV junctional pacemaker activity. In Figure 23-4(A), the P waves have normal configuration and the P-to-P interval is 1.24 sec, corresponding to a regular sinus rhythm at 48 bpm. The QRS complexes have almost an identical rate with normal supraventricular configuration. P waves do not have a regular relationship to the QRS complexes that follow them. The rhythm is intermittent AV dissociation due to SB and passive junctional escape. Note that in this example retrograde conduction of junctional impulses to the atria does not occur. In Figure 23-4(B), the AV junctional pacemaker is accelerated at a rate of 68 bpm, capturing the atria as well as the ventricle. A retrograde P wave follows each QRS complex.

Complete the following sentences:

1. A secondary pacemaker may control heart rhythm when its rate exceeds the rate of the _____ _____ .

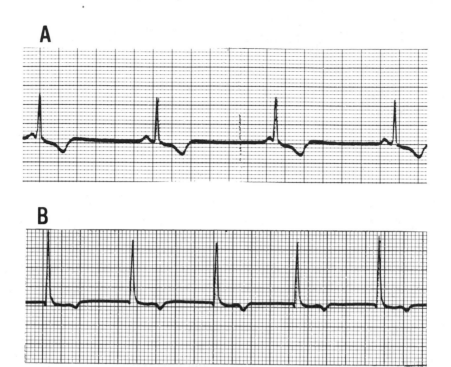

Figure 23-4   AV junctional rhythms; (A) with AV dissociation due to SB and junctional escape, and (B) with retrograde atrial capture during accelerated junction rhythm.

2. During junctional rhythm at 75 bpm, junctional pacing fibers have accelerated to a rate greater than their inherent depolarization rate of _____ to _____ bpm.

3. In Figure 23-5, the pause in heart rhythm lasts for _____ sec and indicates depressed function both of the _____ and of _____ pacemakers.

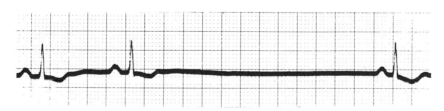

Figure 23-5

4. In Figure 23-6, the SA rate is _____ bpm. The wide QRS complexes have a rate of _____ bpm and represent an _____ pacemaker that has actively accelerated to a rate that transiently competes with sinus rhythm.

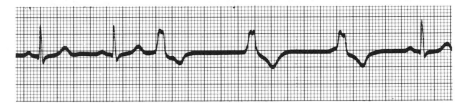

Figure 23-6

Review. Secondary pacemakers that exceed the rate of the SA node may capture the ventricles and also the atria if retrograde conduction occurs. An accelerated junctional focus at 75 bpm exceeds normal junctional pacing rates of 40 to 50 bpm. A 2.8 sec pause would not occur without depression of automaticity both in the SA node and in secondary pacemakers. Figure 23-6 illustrates an accelerated idioventricular rhythm at 55 bpm, competing with sinus rhythm at 69 bpm.

VENTRICULAR PARASYSTOLE

At times, a relatively slow idioventricular pacemaker may not be suppressed as expected by a more rapid coexisting supraventricular rhythm. This condition, termed *parasystole,* is possible if the idioventricular focus is protected from conducted impulses. Depolarization of supraventricular origin does not enter the idioventricular focus or interrupt the timing of its pacing cycle. In Figure 23-7, the wide ectopic

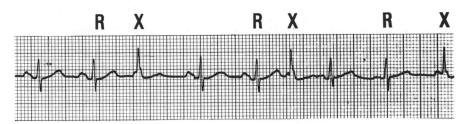

Figure 23-7   Ventricular parasystole.

QRS complexes have no regular relation to the supraventricular QRS complexes that precede them. Note that intervals between idioventricular beats (X) and the preceding sinus beats (R) are completely irregular. The idioventricular beats are related to each other, however, for the intervals between them are constant, 1.8 sec.

Lesson 24

Premature Beats and Tachycardias

Single or repetitive ectopic beats occur ubiquitously. The importance of accurate diagnosis and the frequency of atypical EKG findings mandate careful analysis of this group of rhythm disorders. Choice of arrhythmia therapy may be seriously in error when the EKG interpretation is inaccurate. It is especially important to determine whether an ectopic focus is ventricular or supraventricular.

PREMATURE ATRIAL CONTRACTIONS

EKG features of a typical premature atrial contraction (PAC) are (1) premature P wave that usually differs in configuration from P waves that originate in the SA node, (2) supraventricular QRS complex, and (3) normal or slightly prolonged PRI. Examine Figure 24-1. Two PACs are present. The premature P waves (P′) have identical form indicating unifocal origin. Each P′ wave is followed by a narrow QRS complex. After a PAC, the next sinus beat occurs slightly later than expected. The premature ectopic atrial depolarization enters the SA node and resets the timing of its pacing cycle.

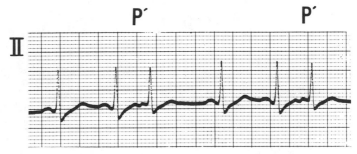

Figure 24-1 Premature atrial contractions.

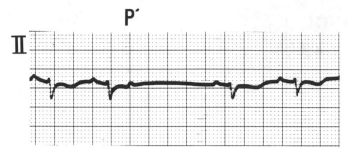

Figure 24-2   Nonconducted PAC.

ATYPICAL PAC WITH DELAYED OR BLOCKED AV CONDUCTION

A PAC that closely follows a normal sinus beat may enter the AV node before the node has returned to normal conductivity. When the AV node is partially or completely refractory, conduction of the PAC to the ventricle may be delayed or completely blocked. In Figure 24-2, the premature P wave (P′) is not followed by a QRS complex. Misinterpretation of nonconducted PACs is common when a T wave obscures the premature P wave, as illustrated in Figure 24-3. The pause in sinus rhythm may be mistaken for SA node dysfunction.

ABERRANT VENTRICULAR CONDUCTION

A common atypical form of PAC is often mistaken for a premature ventricular contraction (PVC) because it displays a wide QRS complex due to delayed, or aberrant, intraventricular conduction as defined in Lesson 13. The premature atrial impulse enters the ventricles before a

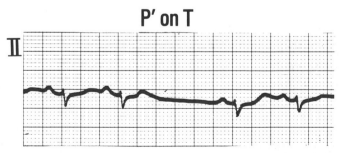

Figure 24-3   Nonconducted PAC with premature P wave obscured by T wave.

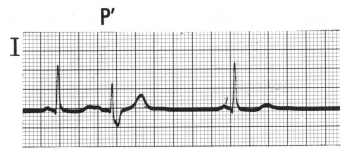

Figure 24-4 PAC with aberrant ventricular conduction resembling a PVC of LV origen, with RBBB configuration of the premature QRS complex.

part of the ventricular conduction system has recovered conductivity. The refractory path, usually the right bundle branch, does not conduct the premature beat, which then shows QRS configuration of RBBB. In Figure 24-4, the second P wave is premature and the wide QRS complex that follows it has a RBBB pattern.

PREMATURE JUNCTIONAL BEATS

Premature junctional beats (PJCs) typically display a narrow supraventricular QRS complex. Like PACs, they also may show a wide QRS due to aberrant ventricular condition. Retrograde P waves may or may not be present.

Complete the following sentences:

1. In Figure 24-5, two PACs are present. The first premature P wave falls in the _____ segment of a SA beat. Because this PAC enters the _____ node before this structure has recovered normal conductivity, its conduction to the _____ is delayed, resulting in a PRI of _____ sec. This PAC also encounters

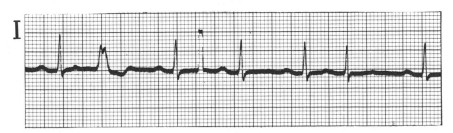

Figure 24-5

a refractory pathway in the _____ bundle branch, resulting in _____ ventricular conduction.

2. Figure 24-6 shows a rapid, irregular rhythm with varying _____ wave configuration, an example of _____ _____ tachycardia, as described in Lesson 10.

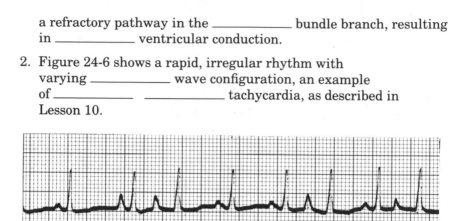

Figure 24-6

3. In Figure 24-7, the atrial rate is _____ bpm. The ventricular rhythm is regular at _____ bpm. This rhythm disorder is _____ _____ with 2:1 AV conduction.

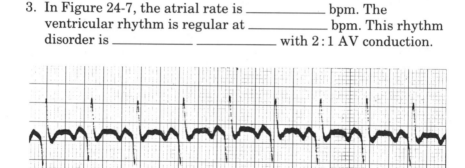

Figure 24-7

Review. The first of two PACs in Figure 24-5 falls in an ST segment. It is delayed in the AV node, with PRI 0.24 sec, and in the left bundle branch. This pattern of aberrant ventricular conduction is somewhat atypical: RBBB is the usual QRS abnormality. The rapid varying P waves of Figure 24-6 illustrate multifocal atrial tachycardia. Alternate atrial waves in Figure 24-7 coincide with QRS complexes, partially obscuring the diagnosis of atrial flutter with 2:1 AV conduction, atrial rate 250 bpm.

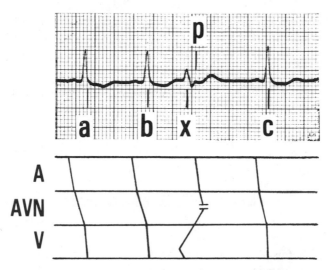

Figure 24-8   PVC (X) with compensatory pause.

PREMATURE VENTRICULAR CONTRACTIONS

In Lesson 14, you learned the principal EKG features of ventricular ectopic beats. These wide QRS beats may resemble a BBB pattern that reflects the ventricle of origin. In contrast to PACs, PVCs ordinarily do not interrupt the pacing cycle of the SA node. As the ladder diagram in Figure 24-8 illustrates, electrical activity from the PVC (x) travels retrograde to the AV node, but is not conducted through the node to the atrium. The atria are paced by the SA node. A P wave lies hidden within the PVC complex. Because regular SA node pacing has not been interrupted, the interval bc that includes the PVC is twice the interval ab of sinus rhythm. Use calipers to verify this relationship. The interval xc is termed a *compensatory pause*. It balances, or compensates for, the short

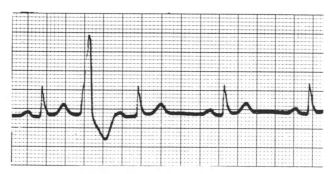

Figure 24-9   Interpolated PVC.

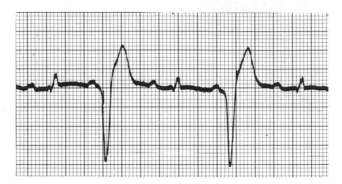

Figure 24-10 Late-diastolic PVCs.

bx interval before the premature beat. The presence of a compensatory pause helps to verify that a premature wide QRS beat is a PVC and not a PAC with aberrant ventricular conduction.

When sinus rhythm is slow, a PVC may occur between sinus beats without a compensatory pause. Figure 24-9 illustrates this atypical form, termed an *interpolated PVC*. A PVC in late diastole may occur during the PR segment and follow a P wave, as shown in Figure 24-10.

Complete the following sentences:

1. In Figure 24-11, lead I shows a wide QRS complex that has _____ bundle branch configuration. It is preceded by

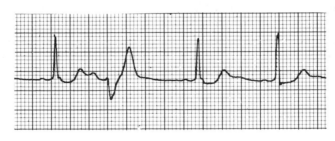

Figure 24-11

   a _____ wave. It is not followed by a _____ pause. This complex represents a _____ with _____ conduction.

2. The wide QRS complex in Figure 24-12 is an _____ _____ . The following complex shows abnormal _____ _____ inversion.

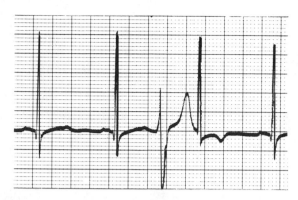

Figure 24-12

Review. Figure 24-11 shows a PAC with aberrant ventricular conduction. The premature P wave is clearly visible and the QRS complex shows typical RBBB configuration. The pause after the premature beat is noncompensatory; the PAC enters the SA node and resets its pacing cycle. The interpolated PVC in Figure 24-12 causes nonspecific T wave inversion for the beat that follows it.

The reentry concept helps to explain many aspects of ventricular arrhythmias. On an individual rhythm strip, unifocal PVCs usually occur at a fixed interval after a supraventricular beat. Examine Figure 24-13. The absence of P waves and the irregular narrow QRS complexes are typical of AF. Three PVCs are present; each follows a supraventricular QRS complex after an interval of 0.44 sec. This paired relationship, or fixed coupling, is typical of reentry. Note that during AF, a PVC is not followed by a compensatory pause, which can occur only during sinus rhythm.

Another phenomenon related to reentry is the *ventricular vulnerable period,* a phase of repolarization that occurs just before the T wave peak. At this stage, ventricular electrical potentials are unevenly distributed because some fibers have repolarized completely while neigh-

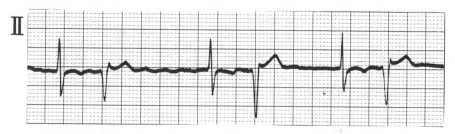

Figure 24-13   PVCs coupled to supraventricular beats during AF.

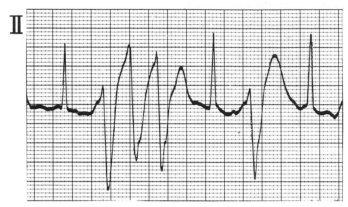

Figure 24-14 PVCs in the ventricular vulnerable period, with reentrant three-beat salvo.

boring fibers have not. This unequal dispersion of electrical potential favors reentry. Experimentally, electrical stimulation of the ventricle during the vulnerable period provokes a series of reentrant ectopic beats. An early PVC that falls in the vulnerable period has a similar capacity to precipitate ventricular tachycardia. In Figure 24-14, a vulnerable period PVC initiates a three-beat salvo.

A related problem concerns occurrence of ventricular arrhythmias when the QTI is prolonged. Recall that QTI duration increases during bradycardia. The QTI may also be prolonged by drugs, or rarely as an inherited trait that may be associated with familial deafness (Jervell and Lange-Nielsen syndrome). All of these conditions may predispose to reentrant ventricular arrhythmias, including ventricular fibrillation (VF).

PVCs are clinically important for two principal reasons. First, they may be an indication of underlying cardiac disease or of drug toxicity.

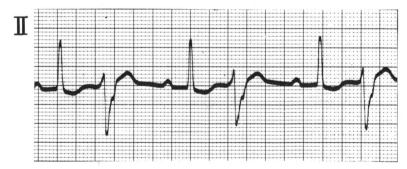

Figure 24-15 Bigeminy due to PVCs.

Second, in patients at special risk, they may have prognostic value regarding the likelihood of a more serious ventricular arrhythmia. In selected clinical settings, four EKG features of PVCs may suggest an increased risk of ventricular tachycardia or VF. These are excessive frequency, multifocal origin, occurrence in pairs or groups, and occurrence during the ventricular vulnerable period (R on T beats).

In Figure 24-15, every other ventricular beat is a PVC. This form of bigeminal rhythm tends to be self-perpetuating (the "rule of bigeminy"). During this rhythm, each SA beat follows a compensatory pause and this pause predisposes to another ventricular reentry cycle.

Complete the following sentences:

1. In Figure 24-16, the interval A corresponds to the _____ period. In certain clinical settings, a PVC that occurs during this interval may result in _____ _____ .

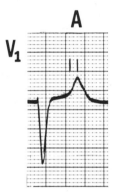

Figure 24-16

2. Figure 24-17 shows two conditions that may predispose to reentrant ventricular arrhythmias. These are _____ and _____ _____ interval.

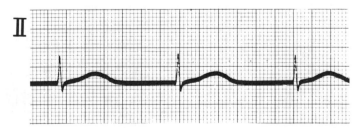

Figure 24-17

3. Figure 24-18 shows _____ PVCs, a form of ventricular warning arrhythmia in selected clinical settings.

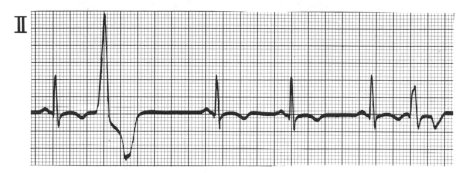

Figure 24-18

Review. Because of dispersed cellular electrical potentials during repolarization, a PVC during the ventricular vulnerable period (A) may precipitate ventricular tachycardia. Bradycardia (48 bpm) and prolonged QTI (0.60 sec), illustrated in Figure 24-17, may predispose to reentrant ventricular arrhythmias. Multifocal PVCs, illustrated in Figure 24-18, may indicate increased risk of ventricular tachycardia in certain patients.

VENTRICULAR TACHYCARDIA

Ventricular tachycardia may complicate many diseases that affect ventricular muscle. In acute CAD or in advanced ventricular failure, ventricular tachycardia is commonly life threatening. Diagnosis of this arrhythmia must often be made under emergency conditions. The EKG may show single or repetitive groups of rapid wide QRS complexes, often with a slightly irregular rhythm, as illustrated in Figure 24-19. Sustained ventricular tachycardia usually has a nearly regular rate between 140 and 200 bpm. QRS duration often exceeds 0.14 sec and

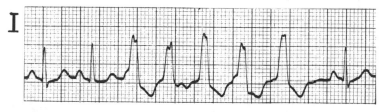

Figure 24-19   Five-beat episode of ventricular tachycardia, rate 150 bpm.

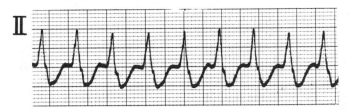

Figure 24-20 Sustained ventricular tachycardia, rate 155 bpm.

marked LAD is commonly present. Figure 24-20 illustrates ventricular tachycardia at 155 bpm. Secondary ST and T wave abnormalities are prominent.

In Lesson 13, you learned that supraventricular beats may display wide QRS complexes because of a chronic BBB, because of a temporary BBB pattern (AVC), or because of conduction through an AV bypass tract (WPW syndrome). Supraventricular tachycardias with wide QRS complexes must be distinguished from ventricular tachycardia. A key step in this differential diagnosis is to discover whether the atrial and ventricular rhythms are independent of each other, a form of AV dissociation that occurs in about one-half of patients with ventricular tachycardia.

Examine Figure 24-21, an example of wide QRS tachycardia. The ventricular rate is 130 bpm and regular. P waves are present at a rate of 88 bpm, although many of them are obscured by ventricular waves. Their timing has no relation to QRS complexes. AV dissociation is present, indicating that the wide QRS beats are not of supraventricular origin and confirming the diagnosis of ventricular tachycardia.

When the atrium has an independent rhythm during ventricular tachycardia, especially if the ventricular rate is not extremely fast, a

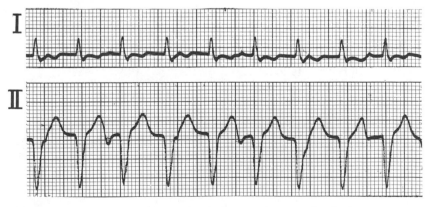

Figure 24-21 Ventricular tachycardia, 140 bpm, with AV dissociation.

supraventricular impulse may occasionally enter the ventricle. During ventricular tachycardia, an occasional narrow QRS or ventricular fusion beat is indirect evidence that AV dissociation is present.

Analysis of wide QRS tachycardia requires the following steps:

1. Search for P waves. Compare adjacent ventricular complexes for deformity caused by superimposed P waves. Occasionally, pervenous insertion of a right atrial electrode may be indicated to identify the atrial rhythm.
2. Examine the QRS complex. Marked widening or extreme LAD favors diagnosis of ventricular tachycardia. RBBB configuration may favor AVC of a supraventricular tachycardia.
3. Search for occasional changes in QRS configuration consistent with ventricular fusion beats.

Complete the following sentences:

1. In Figure 24-22, _____ waves are present at a rate of _____ bpm and each is followed by a _____ that is _____ sec wide. This wide QRS rhythm is _____ tachycardia with _____ .

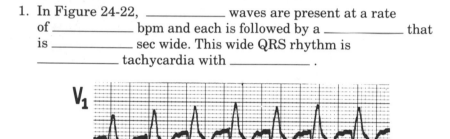

Figure 24-22

2. _____ waves are absent in Figure 24-23 and the totally irregular ventricular rhythm suggests ____·_____ with wide QRS complexes due to _____ .

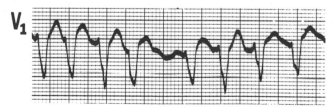

Figure 24-23

3. The wide, bizarre waves in Figure 24-24 are an example of EKG _____ .

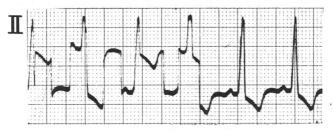

Figure 24-24

Review. Figure 24-22 shows ST with RBBB, rate 135 bpm, QRS duration 0.14 sec. In Figure 24-23, the rhythm is AF with LBBB. Figure 24-24 illustrates EKG artifacts.

Another EKG finding often helps to identify wide QRS beats due to aberrant conduction, especially when the underlying rhythm is AF. AVC tends to occur after a short R-to-R interval that follows a long R-to-R interval (Ashman's phenomenon). The long interval results in a prolonged refractory period for ventricular conduction paths, especially the RBB. In Figure 24-25, the basic rhythm is AF. The three wide QRS complexes are aberrantly conducted beats with RBBB configuration. They develop after a short R-to-R interval (BC) that follows a long interval (AB).

A distinctive form of ventricular tachycardia may occur in certain patients who have prolonged QTI. In this disorder rapid wide QRS complexes change constantly in configuration. Because groups of these complexes alternately point up or down, this multiform ventricular tachycardia has been termed *torsade de pointes,* or twisting of the

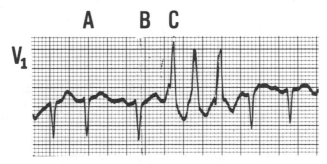

Figure 24-25 Atrial fibrillation with wide QRS beats due to aberrant ventricular conduction, illustrating the Ashman's phenomenon.

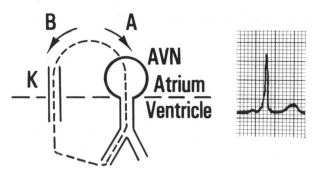

Figure 24-26 Potential pathway for atrioventricular reentrant tachycardia in WPW syndrome, involving the AV node (AVN) and bundle of Kent (K).

points. This arrhythmia may be an outcome of quinidine toxicity in patients who develop marked QT prolongation from this drug.

In Lesson 13, you learned the EKG features of the WPW syndrome, another cause of wide QRS complexes. In this syndrome, impulses from the SA node, or atrial ectopic impulses, enter the ventricles through an accessory conduction bundle that bypasses the AV node. A delta wave represents early excitation of a ventricular segment. The resulting abnormal QRS complex may be only slightly deformed, or the delta wave may cause a large, bizarre complex that is typically peaked and somewhat symmetric ("Eiffel Tower complex"). When AFl or AF occurs in a WPW patient, delta waves may result in wide QRS tachycardia resembling ventricular tachycardia.

Figure 24-26 diagrams an anomalous AV conduction path, or Kent bundle. This path, together with the normal conduction system, forms a potential reentry circuit, illustrated by a dotted line. During a reentrant tachycardia, depolarization may travel either clockwise (arrow A) or counterclockwise (arrow B) around this circuit. A clockwise impulse

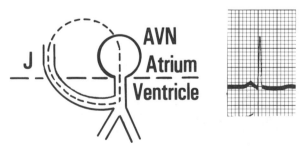

Figure 24-27 AV node bypass due to a James fiber (J) connecting the atrium directly to the His bundle. The corresponding EKG complex displays a short PR interval with normal QRS configuration.

in this illustration will enter the ventricles through the His–Purkinje system and resulting QRS complexes will not be deformed by a delta wave.

Another form of AV bypass tract may cause ventricular preexcitation with normal QRS configuration. Figure 24-27 diagrams a paranodal tract, or James fiber, that connects the atrium to the His bundle rather than directly to the ventricular wall as the Kent bundle does. An atrial impulse conducted rapidly through such a tract is not delayed in the AV node and a short PRI results. This impulse enters the ventricle through normal His–Purkinje pathways and the resulting QRS complex is normal. The paranodal tract also offers a potential conduction circuit for reentrant tachycardia. The occurrence of reentrant supraventricular tachycardias in patients who have a short PRI and normal QRS complex during sinus rhythm constitutes the Lown-Ganong-Levine syndrome.

Lesson 25

Nodal and Infranodal Atrioventricular Block

Conduction of atrial impulses to the ventricles may be interrupted either in the AV node or in structures below the node. The causes, clinical implications, and EKG manifestations of AV block at these two sites differ. AV node conduction may be impaired by vagus nerve stimulation, by drugs, or as a consequence of inferior wall myocardial infarction. These causes are ordinarily reversible. Infranodal block most commonly results from fibrosis of the His-Purkinje system, or rarely accompanies extensive septal infarction. The His bundle electrogram technique discussed in Lesson 7 has been instrumental in clarifying many issues related to the site of AV block.

Classically, three degrees of AV block have been defined.

1. *First degree.* The PRI is prolonged. The AV conduction ratio is 1:1. The AV node is the usual site of this conduction delay.
2. *Second degree.* During sinus rhythm, some atrial impulses are not conducted to the ventricles. Second degree AV block must not be confused with nonconduction of rapid atrial impulses as seen in AFl with 2:1 conduction, a normal function of the AV node.
3. *Third degree.* AV conduction is totally interrupted. Regardless of the atrial rhythm, which may be normal or abnormal, the ventricles have a totally independent regular escape rhythm at a slower rate.

Complete the following sentences:

1. Figure 25-1 shows _____ ° AV block with PRI of _____ sec, reflecting conduction delay in the _____ _____ .

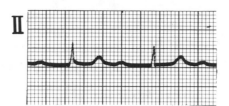

Figure 25-1

2. In Figure 25-2, the first PRI is _____ sec. The second PRI is _____ sec, reflecting AV conduction delay following premature _____ depolarization.

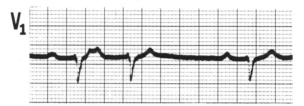

Figure 25-2

3. Because the PRI in Figure 25-3 is _____ sec, the small P waves might not be recognized. This supraventricular rhythm with rate _____ bpm might then be mistakenly diagnosed as _____ _____ rhythm.

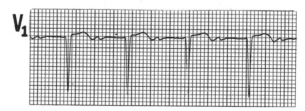

Figure 25-3

Review. In Figure 25-1, delayed AV node conduction is the cause of first degree AV block, with a constant PRI of 0.36 sec. Figure 25-2 shows a PRI of 0.28 sec. A premature P wave is present in the ST segment of the first complex. The PAC shows extreme PR prolongation to 0.42 scc. The PRI in Figure 25-3 is 0.32 sec. Because the P waves are small, this rhythm might be misinterpreted as accelerated junctional rhythm, 85 bpm.

Second degree AV block in the AV node (type I) typically results in progressive widening of the PRI for a series of beats that precede a nonconducted beat. Conduction fails gradually, rather than all at once. Figure 25-4 illustrates this pattern, called the *Wenckebach phenomenon*. Note first that the atrial rhythm is regular; the nonconducted beats are not PACs. The AV conduction ratio is stable at 3 : 2. The PRI increases from 0.20 to 0.28 sec. After the nonconducted beat, the PRI returns to 0.20 sec. The cycle of progressive increase in the PRI then repeats. At times, the AV conduction ratio may change from cycle to cycle. The conduction ratio during type I second degree AV block is usually 3 : 2 or 4 : 3, but cycles of progressive AV node conduction failure may be much longer.

Infranodal second degree AV block (Mobitz type, or type II) reflects an abrupt conduction failure. The PRI is the same for all conducted beats. Figure 25-5 illustrates this rare pattern. With second degree infranodal AV block, because the underlying disease or degenerative process almost invariably involves the bundle branches, QRS complexes will show BBB.

Note that for second degree AV block with 2-to-1 conduction, the Wenckebach phenomenon cannot be identified. There is no opportunity

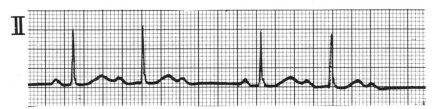

Figure 25-4   Second degree AV nodal block (type I) with Wenckebach phenomenon.

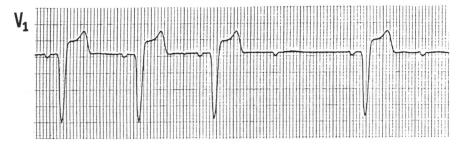

Figure 25-5   Second degree infranodal block (type II or Mobitz type). The PRI is 0.16 sec for each conducted atrial beat. QRS duration is 0.14 sec because of coexisting BBB.

to observe progressive widening of the PRI. If the QRS complexes are normal during 2:1 conduction, the site of block is probably in the AV node.

Third degree block in the AV node typically results in a junctional escape rhythm. QRS complexes show a narrow supraventricular configuration unless they are wide because of coexisting BBB. The ventricular rate is usually 40 to 50 bpm and regular. Examine Figure 25-6. Seven P waves are present at a slightly irregular rate near 75 bpm. The narrow supraventricular QRS complexes have a regular rate of 48 bpm that is totally independent of the atrial rhythm.

Infranodal third degree AV block results in a slow idioventricular escape rhythm, usually at a rate near 35 bpm, with wide QRS complexes.

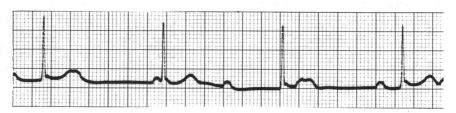

Figure 25-6 Third degree AV nodal block with junctional escape rhythm.

Recall that slow ventricular rates promote reentrant ventricular ectopic beats. Third degree AV block may be complicated by PVCs or ventricular tachycardia. In this setting, either ventricular tachycardia or ventricular asystole may cause syncopal attacks (Stokes-Adams syncope).

Complete the following sentences:

1. In Figure 25-7 the atrial rate is _____ bpm, with _____ -to- _____ AV conduction. Because the QRS complex is _____ sec in duration, the site of _____ degree AV block could be intranodal.

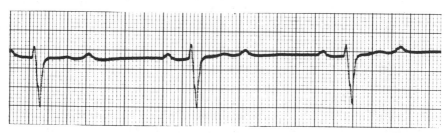

Figure 25-7

2. Figure 25-8 shows an atrial wave pattern typical of _____. The supraventricular QRS complexes are regular at _____ bpm, independent of atrial rhythm, indicating _____ degree AV block at the level of the _____ _____.

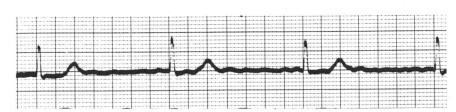

Figure 25-8

3. In Figure 25-9, atrial arrest is associated with an abnormally slow _____ escape rhythm.

4. Ventricular rate in Figure 25-10 is regular at _____ bpm, with QRS duration of _____ sec, indicating _____ degree AV block at the _____ level.

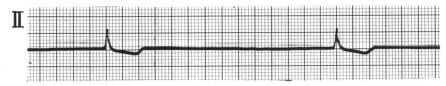

Figure 25-9

Review. Figure 25-7 illustrates second degree AV block with 2 : 1 conduction, which could be infranodal with QRS duration 0.14 sec, atrial rate 71 bpm. In Figure 25-8, AF is associated with third degree

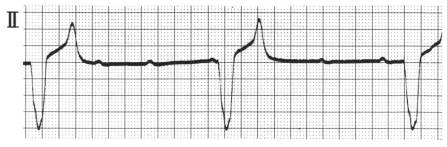

Figure 25-10

block in the AV node and junctional escape rhythm at 43 bpm. Figure 25-9 shows no evidence of atrial activity and an abnormally slow junctional escape rhythm. In Figure 25-10, third degree infranodal block results in an idioventricular escape rhythm at 26 bpm, with QRS duration 0.22 sec.

Lesson 26

Artificial Pacemakers

Pacemaker design has become increasingly sophisticated and potential problems in EKG interpretation of paced rhythms have increased accordingly. A standard letter code for pacemaker functions is:

Chamber paced or sensed

A = atrium

V = ventricle

D = both chambers (dual)

O = no sensing function

Pacemaker response to sensed spontaneous beats

I = inhibited

T = triggered

D = inhibited or triggered

A combination of three letters describes basic features of each pacing mode. A VVI unit, for example, paces the ventricles. It also senses spontaneous ventricular beats, which inhibit the pulse generator output. This unit paces only "on demand." When a spontaneous rhythm is present at a ventricular rate faster than the pacemaker's rate, the pulse generator is inactive. Pacing resumes if the spontaneous rhythm stops or slows excessively. VVI pacemakers are particularly suitable for many patients who have symptoms due to intermittent bradycardia, as seen with severe SA node dysfunction or with intermittent advanced AV block and slow ventricular escape rhythm.

Examine Figure 26-1. P waves are regular at 69 bpm; they have no consistent relation to ventricular complexes. Pacing artifacts are regular at 73 bpm, each followed by a QRS complex that is wide and bizarre because of ectopic origin of ventricular depolarization. Ventricular activation begins at the point where the pacing electrode contacts the

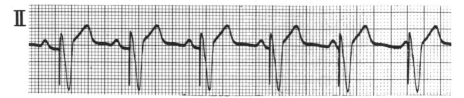

Figure 26-1   Advanced AV block with paced ventricular rhythm (VOO).

ventricular wall. AV dissociation is present; the SA node controls the atria and the pacemaker controls the ventricles. Figure 26-1 illustrates fixed-rate ventricular pacing (VOO).

Pacing artifacts may be positive, negative, or biphasic. Their display on the EKG does not depend on proper placement of the pacing electrode. Pacing artifacts continue to appear in spite of abnormal electrode tip position in the superior vena cava or in the pericardium following ventricular perforation. Under these circumstances, the artifacts are not followed by QRS complexes because the pacemaker fails to capture the ventricles.

Examine Figure 26-2. P waves are not visible; the patient has AF with low-amplitude fibrillation waves. The third QRS complex is a spontaneous ventricular beat. Note that this beat interrupts the regular pacing artifacts, which resume after an interval of 0.88 sec. This time lapse, termed the *pacemaker escape interval,* is longer than the regular pacing interval of 0.83 sec. Sensing and pacing functions of this VVI pacemaker are intact. The spontaneous ventricular beat inhibits the pulse generator, and every pacing impulse captures ventricular contraction.

Complete the following sentences:

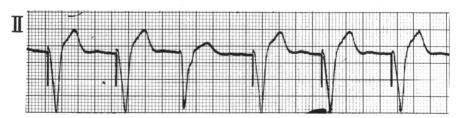

Figure 26-2   AF with paced ventricular rhythm on demand (VVI).

1. In Figure 26-3, the first QRS complex is narrow, an indication that depolarization enters the ventricles through the _____ , not from the pacing electrode. Because the second pacing impulse captures a part of the ventricle, the QRS complex that follows it is characteristic of a _____ beat. During paced beats the lead I QRS complexes resemble _____ BBB, an indication that the pacing electrode lies in the _____ ventricle.

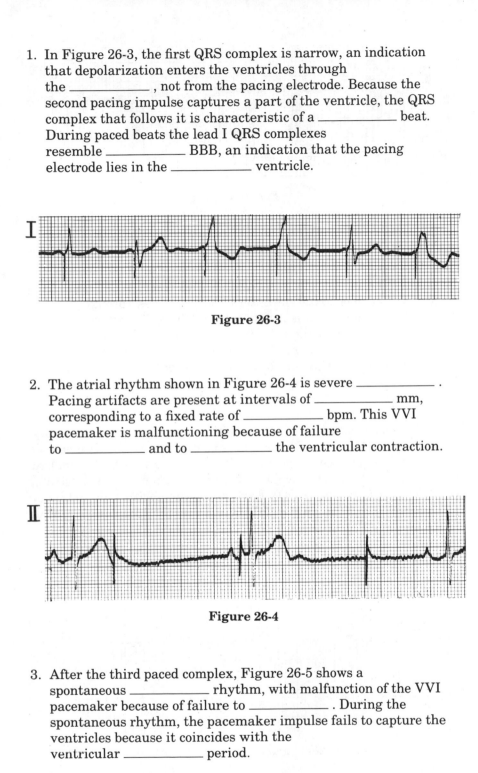

Figure 26-3

2. The atrial rhythm shown in Figure 26-4 is severe _____ . Pacing artifacts are present at intervals of _____ mm, corresponding to a fixed rate of _____ bpm. This VVI pacemaker is malfunctioning because of failure to _____ and to _____ the ventricular contraction.

Figure 26-4

3. After the third paced complex, Figure 26-5 shows a spontaneous _____ rhythm, with malfunction of the VVI pacemaker because of failure to _____ . During the spontaneous rhythm, the pacemaker impulse fails to capture the ventricles because it coincides with the ventricular _____ period.

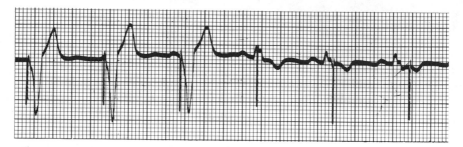

Figure 26-5

Review. The initial supraventricular QRS complex of Figure 26-3 indicates that depolarization enters the ventricles through the His bundle. The second QRS is a fusion beat. The QRS pattern of LBBB during pacing implies right ventricular origin of depolarization. In Figure 26-4, the pacemaker fails to sense and capture during severe SB. The pacing interval of 38 mm (152 msec) corresponds to a rate of 40 bpm (1500 divided by 38). In Figure 26-5, the pacemaker fails to sense the presence of sinus rhythm and does not capture the ventricles during the refractory period.

When AV conduction is intact, patients with symptomatic bradycardia due to SA node dysfunction may be candidates for atrial pacing. In contrast to ventricular pacing, this mode preserves the normal sequence of atrial and ventricular contractions. Figure 26-6 illustrates fixed-rate atrial pacing (AOO). Each pacing artifact is followed by an abnormal P wave. The PRI is 0.20 sec and the QRS complexes are wide because of IVCD.

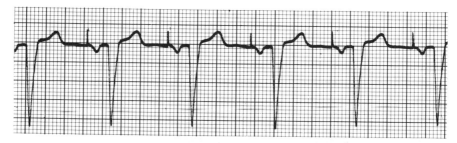

Figure 26-6   Paced atrial rhythm (AOO).

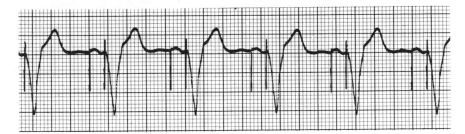

Figure 26-7   AV sequential paced rhythm (DVI).

Figure 26-7 illustrates AV sequential pacing (DVI). For each cycle, two pacing artifacts are present, the first followed by a P wave and the second by a wide QRS complex. Like VVI units, pacemakers in this node are inhibited by spontaneous ventricular contractions.

7 | EKG Syndromes

Lesson 27

Myocardial Infarction

In previous lessons, you have learned the typical effects of myocardial infarction upon the QRS complex, ST segment, and T wave. Table 27-1 summarizes these effects and their chronological sequence of evolution. Routine leads are well positioned to display these abnormalities when infarction is in the anteroseptal or inferior left ventricular wall. With posterior wall infarction, leads V_1 and V_2 record abnormal waves that are opposite in direction to the Q waves, elevated ST segments, and inverted T waves typically seen with anterior wall infarction. The pathophysiology of coronary artery disease is complex and variations are commonplace from the typical infarction patterns listed in Table 27.1.

For initial infarcts, the EKG lead group involved correlates well with the site of coronary occlusion and location of infarction. Right coronary artery occlusion is the usual cause of inferior wall infarction, at times with posterior wall involvement. Occlusion of the left anterior descending artery is the cause of septal and anterior wall infarction. Infarction due to left circumflex occlusion may be confined to the pos-

Table 27-1 Evolution of EKG Abnormalities Due to Uncomplicated Transmural Myocardial Infarction

Stage of Infarction and Time Interval After Onset	Typical EKG Abnormalities in Principal Leads Affected
Immediate or hyperacute (minutes to hours)	ST segment elevated T wave amplitude increased
Acute (hours to days)	Q waves progressively wider and deeper ST segment gradually less elevated T waves progressively more deeply inverted
Late or convalescent (days to months)	Q waves stable or gradually normalized ST segment normal T wave gradually less inverted or normalized

terior wall. Accuracy of anatomic correlations diminishes when old or recent infarcts are present at multiple sites.

Figure 27-1 illustrates the typical effects of inferior wall infarction 6 hours (A) and 3 days (B) after onset. Note that large Q waves develop promptly in this example. At 6 hours, ST elevation in the inferior leads is accompanied by reciprocal ST depression in lead aVL.

Figure 27-2 shows evidence of both posterior wall infarction and inferior wall infarction. Wide Q waves in the inferior leads and tall R waves in leads V_1 and V_2 indicate transmural involvement. Both the inferior lead ST elevation and the ST depression in V_1–V_3 are manifestations of acute injury.

In Figure 27-3, the precordial leads illustrate QRS abnormalities of old anterior infarction, (A) and old posterior wall infarction (B). Note that Q wave evidence of the anterior infarct is not distinct, but reversed R wave progression is present, with R V_2 taller than R V_{3-4}. For the posterior infarct, the wide R wave in V_1 may be considered a *Q wave equivalent*. It exceeds 0.04 sec in duration. For both patterns, the leads with QRS abnormalities show no distinct ST or T wave abnormalities at this late, or fully evolved, stage.

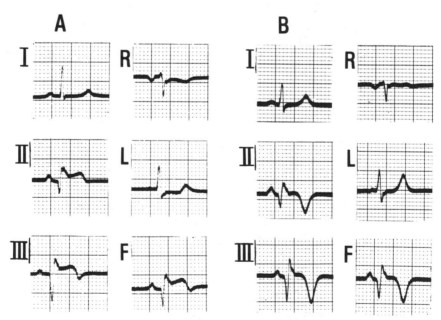

Figure 27-1   Effects of acute inferior myocardial infarction in limb leads, (A) 6 hours and (B) 3 days after onset.

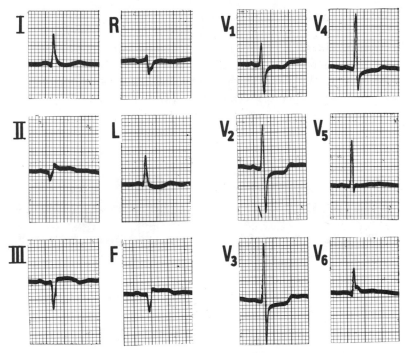

Figure 27-2 Effects of inferior and posterior myocardial infarction, acute stage.

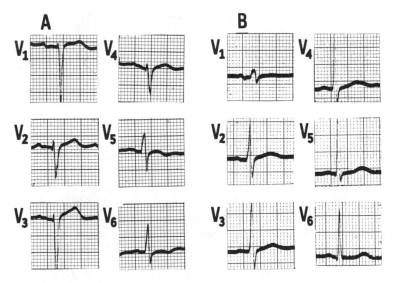

Figure 27-3 Effects of (A) anterior and (B) posterior myocardial infarction in chest leads.

Complete the following sentences:

1. In Figure 27-4(A), ST _____ extends from lead
_____ to lead _____ , and _____
amplitude is increased. These are typical manifestations of
anterior myocardial infarction during the _____ stage,
_____ to _____ after onset.

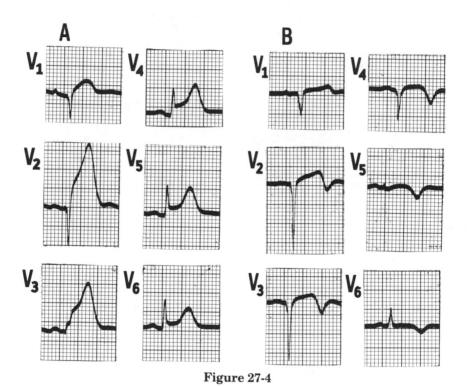

Figure 27-4

2. The ventricular depolarization complexes in Figure 27-4(B)
have _____ configuration in leads V_1 through V_4,
indicating that the anterior infarction is transmural. The ST-T
wave abnormalities suggest that infarction occurred
_____ to _____ before the tracing was recorded.

3. Figure 27-5, the emergency room tracing of a 50-year-old man
with severe chest pain shows _____ .

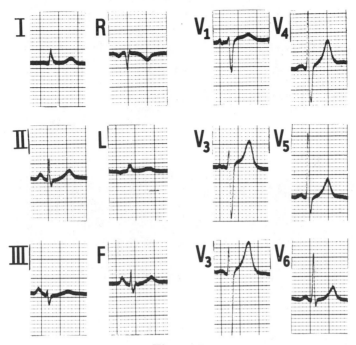

Figure 27-5

Review. ST elevation and increased T wave amplitude in leads V_1 through V_6 of Figure 27-4(A) are immediate or hyperacute abnormalities, which may be present minutes to a few hours after acute anterior myocardial infarction. The QS complexes of Figure 27-4(B) indicate transmural infarction. This tracing, recorded on the third postinfarct day, shows acute stage ST and T wave abnormalities that may be seen hours or days after the event. Figure 27-5 is a normal EKG that does not exclude acute coronary artery disease as the cause of chest pain.

Atypical or complicated EKG manifestations of myocardial infarction occur frequently. Figure 27-6 illustrates inferior wall infarction complicated by LBBB. When LBBB is present, Q wave criteria for infarction may be invalid. LBBB alters initial QRS forces and commonly results in QS complexes in anteroseptal leads. Patients with LBBB, however, may develop ST-T wave evidence of acute infarction, as seen in Figure 27-6(A). After 2 weeks, in Figure 27-6(B), ST elevation in the inferior leads has diminished and T wave inversion is present. After 18 months, in Figure 27-6(C), LBBB has resolved and lead III shows a QS complex consistent with old infarction.

Figure 27-7 illustrates evolution of an atypical anterolateral in-

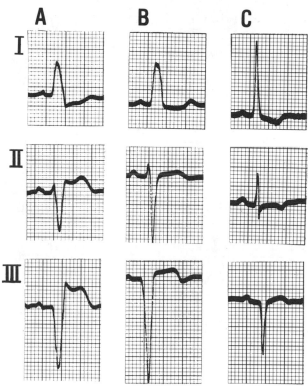

A **B** **C**

I

II

III

Figure 27-6 Effects of inferior myocardial infarction on standard limb leads
in presence of LBBB, (A) immediately, (B) after 2 weeks, and
(C) after 18 months.

farction. In comparison to a preinfarction EKG (A), the acute stage
tracing (B) shows ST elevation and more prominent Q waves. Subsequent tracings at 7 days (C) and 17 days (D) show progressive T wave
inversion without Q waves, a pattern often associated with non-
transmural infarction. Transient Q waves may reflect loss of electrical
forces from a reversibly ischemic or "stunned" segment of the LV wall.

Complete the following sentences:

1. In Figure 27-8, ST elevation in leads _____ , _____ ,
   and V₁ through V₅ indicate acute
   _____ infarction, with _____ ST depression in
   inferior leads. Q waves are present in spite of _____ BBB.
   In the frontal plane, initial QRS forces show prominent
   _____ axis deviation as seen with left _____
   _____ block.

2. In Figure 27-9, Q waves are accompanied by ST segment

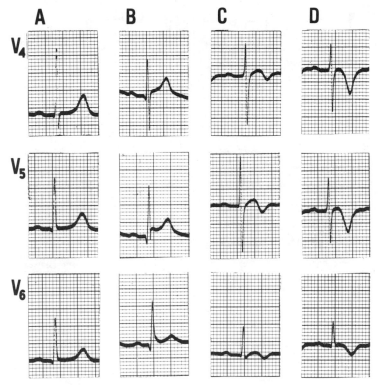

Figure 27-7 Effects of atypical anterolateral myocardial infarction, (B) immediately, (C) after 7 days, and (D) after 17 days.

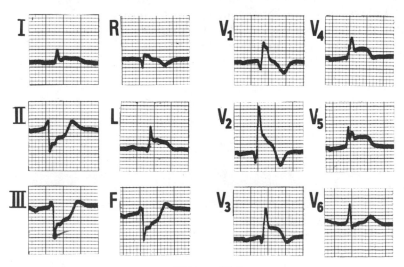

Figure 27-8

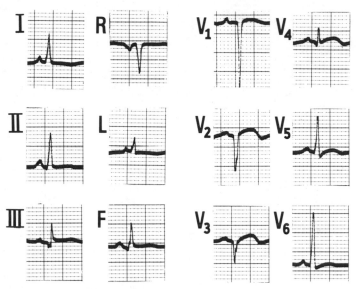

Figure 27-9

_____ consistent with recent infarction or with old infarction complicated by _____ _____.

Review. The acute anteroseptal infarction pattern in Figure 27-8 has typical Q waves and ST elevation inspite of RBBB and left anterior fascicular block. ST elevation in I and aVL is accompanied by reciprocal inferior lead ST depression. Infarction in Figure 27-9 may be recent, but the ST elevation is also consistent with a chronic pattern due to ventricular aneurysm. Involvement of both anterior and inferior lead groups commonly indicates infarction of the LV apex.

Lesson 28

Ventricular Hypertrophy

In Lessons 15, 19, and 22, you learned the individual EKG effects of ventricular hypertrophy. For LVH, these are high QRS voltage, IVCD, LAD, downsloping ST segment depression, and T wave inversion. Typically these abnormalities are most prominent in anterolateral leads. In older patients, high QRS voltage is the most sensitive criterion. Individually, each finding is nonspecific. Patient age, chest wall thickness, and other influences have important effects on QRS amplitude. When ST-T wave abnormalities are present, they may have causes other than LVH, especially digitalis effect. LAD generally reflects conduction system fibrosis that is only indirectly related to ventricular hypertrophy.

The EKG diagnosis of LVH offers many pitfalls. Useful conclusions depend on recognition of combinations of abnormal findings and on their clinical context. Remember that the pathophysiology of LVH is complex. In addition, common coexisting disorders, especially CAD and conduction system fibrosis, have major EKG effects that obscure or mimic LVH patterns. At times, the EKG may be entirely normal when major anatomic LVH is present.

For systematic application of LVH criteria, Romhilt and Estes devised a scale that ranks EKG findings according to their correlation with LV weight at autopsy. Table 28-1 is a modified version of this scale. It can be applied by a minimally trained technician or by a computer. It is a useful background for analysis of an individual EKG, but should not be used inflexibly. Such scales clearly have limitations. They have no reference to clinical context. They do not distinguish between minimal and marked increases in QRS amplitude or between typical and atypical ST-T wave abnormalities.

Figure 28-1 illustrates an LVH pattern in the EKG of a 45-year-old patient with hypertension. R wave amplitude in V_5 is 33 mm, or 3.3 mV. Typical T wave abnormalities are present in anterolateral leads. The QRS axis is $-30°$. QRS duration measured in the limb leads is 0.09 sec, and lead I shows intrinsicoid deflection of 0.04 sec. An LAE pattern is not evident. The total point score of 8 corresponds to LVH.

Figure 28-2 illustrates atypical features of LVH in the EKG of a 33-year-old man with severe valvular aortic stenosis. Leads III and a

Table 28-1 Scale of EKG Abnormalities Associated with LVH in Older Adults at Autopsy

Score	EKG Abnormality
3	High QRS voltage: limb lead R or S > 2.0 mV V_{1-2} S > 3.0 mV V_{5-6} R > 3.0 mV S V_{1-2} + R V_{5-6} > 4.0 mV
3	ST depression and/or T wave inversion in leads with tall R wave (without digitalis)
2	LAD (QRS axis − 30 to −90°)
1	QRS duration ⩾ 0.09 sec in limb lead, or intrinsicoid deflection ⩾ 0.05 sec
(3)	LAE (in absence of mitral valve disease)

Interpretation of total score: ⩾ 6—LVH
 5—probable LVH
 4—possible LVH

VF show abnormal Q waves, and R waves are absent in leads V_1 through V_4, a prominent pseudoinfarction pattern. In this patient, infarction was not evident at autopsy. This EKG also shows marked anterolateral ST depression and T wave inversion, with reciprocal ST elevation in V_1 and V_2. S wave amplitude in V_2 is 4.4 mV and QRS duration is 0.10 sec measured in lead I or a VL. Note the calibration artifact, 1 mV = 0.5 cm.

Complete the following sentences:

1. For Figure 28.3, the routine EKG of a 40-year-old man, the single lead that shows the most definite evidence of LVH is _____ . The total LVH point score for this tracing is _____ .

2. Pseudoinfarction patterns due to LVH consist of _____ waves or waves with _____ configuration that may mimic infarction of the _____ , inferior, or anterolateral zones of the LV wall.

Review. High QRS voltage, the most definite EKG criterion for LVH, is most prominent in the 4.0-mV S wave of lead V_2, Figure 28-3 (1 mV = 0.05 cm). High QRS voltage, QRS duration of 0.10 sec, and ST-T wave abnormalities account for an LVH score of seven points. Q or QS waves due to LVH may mimic inferior or anteroseptal infarcts as evident in Figure 28-2.

RVH patterns are often misinterpreted, in part because they are uncommon. Tall R waves in lead V_1 are an important manifestation,

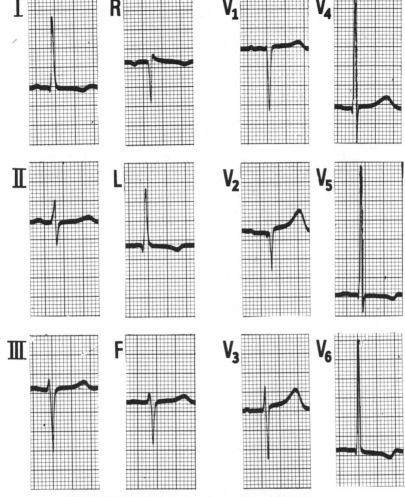

Figure 28-1 Typical effects of LVH.

but other causes for this finding include counterclockwise rotation, posterior wall infarction, RBBB, and WPW syndrome. In older patients, RAD is a useful clue to RVH, although this finding also has other causes such as left posterior fascicular block. Table 28-2 summarizes the most common EKG findings associated with RVH in adults.

Examine Figure 28-4. The R wave in lead V_1 with normal QRS duration of 0.08 sec is typical evidence of moderately severe RVH. V_6 displays a prominent S wave. The QRS axis is +90°. An RV strain pattern is present, with ST-T wave abnormalities in both the right precordial lead group and the inferior leads. P wave abnormalities of

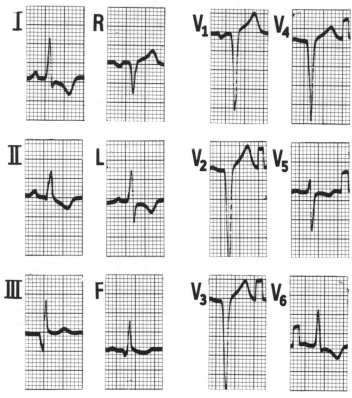

Figure 28-2 Atypical effects of LVH, with prominent pseudoinfarction pattern.

LAE suggest the diagnosis of mitral stenosis with RVH due to pulmonary hypertension.

Complete the following sentences:

1. Figure 28-5 shows a tall _____ wave in lead V_1 and wide _____ wave in lead I, with QRS duration of _____ due to _____ .

2. In Figure 28-6, _____ axis deviation is present. T wave inversion is present in leads V_5 and V_6, an atypical finding for _____ hypertrophy. P wave amplitude is _____ mm in lead II, indicating _____ .

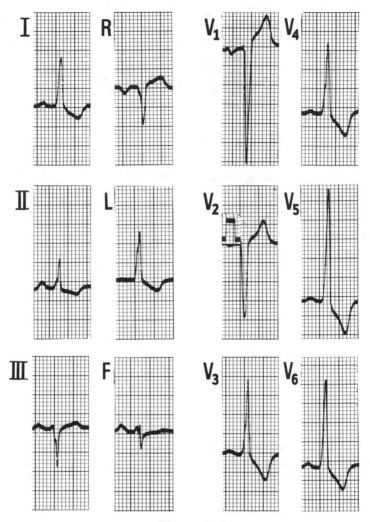

Figure 28-3

Table 28-2 Principal EKG Effects of RVH

QRS complex	V_1: R > S
	qR or R
	rSR′ with tall R′
	V_6: deep S wave
	RAD
ST segment	Depressed ⎰ in V_{1-3} and/or
T wave	Inverted ⎱ II, III, aVF

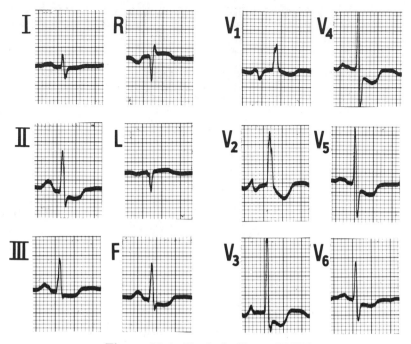

Figure 28-4　Typical effects of RVH.

Review. In Figure 28-5, QRS duration is 0.14 sec. The wide R wave in V_1 and S wave in lead I are typical of RBBB. Figure 28-6 shows marked RAD with QRS axis near +140°, in the positive sector for a VR on the hexaxial reference diagram. T wave inversion in V_5 and V_6 is not a typical manifestation of RVH. In lead II, P wave amplitude of 3.5 mm is evidence of RAE.

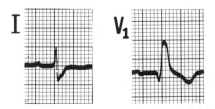

Figure 28-5

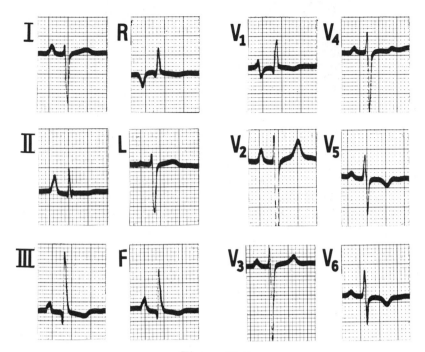

Figure 28-6

Lesson 29

Acute Cor Pulmonale

The leading cause of acute cor pulmonale is massive pulmonary embolism. EKG abnormalities aid in this important diagnosis, but are of little help in diagnosis of smaller pulmonary emboli that do not cause pulmonary hypertension. Table 29-1 lists EKG manifestations of acute cor pulmonale, which may occur individually or in various combinations. They are typically transient, resolving over a period of hours or days as pulmonary hypertension subsides. When Q waves and T wave inversion appear in lead III, the pattern may mimic inferior wall myocardial infarction.

Figure 29-1(A) illustrates limb lead abnormalities in a 28-year-old patient with sudden dyspnea and hypotension during convalescence from knee surgery. The $S_I Q_{III}$ pattern is accompanied by ST and T wave abnormalities. In Figure 29-1(B), an EKG taken 4 days later, these abnormalities have resolved.

Complete the following sentence:

1. In Figure 29-2, the QRS axis is _____ and _____ rotation is present. There is evidence of _____ enlargement. In an appropriate clinical setting, these findings are consistent with _____ _____ .

Table 29-1 EKG Effects of Acute Cor Pulmonale

P wave	RAE
QRS complex	RAD
	Clockwise rotation
	RBBB
	$S_I Q_{III}$
	$S_I S_{II} S_{III}$
ST segment	Depressed ⎰ in V_{1-3} and/or
T wave	Inverted ⎱ II, III, aVF

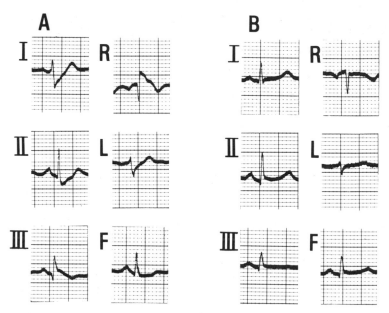

Figure 29-1 Acute cor pulmonale, (A) immediately and (B) 4 days after acute pulmonary embolism.

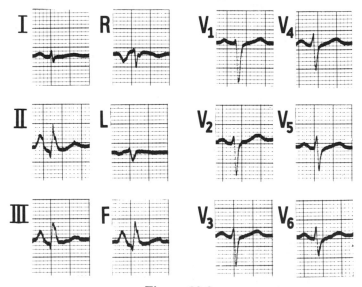

Figure 29-2

Review. The vertical QRS axis of 90° in Figure 29-2, clockwise rotation and RAE are consistent with acute cor pulmonale.

Lesson 30

Cardiomyopathy

Heart muscle diseases include a wide variety of anatomic abnormalities and their EKG manifestations are equally varied. Clinical diagnosis of these disorders is often difficult. Hypertrophic cardiomyopathy, an idiopathic and commonly familial condition, may cause asymmetric hypertrophy involving principally the ventricular septum. Dilated, or congestive, cardiomyopathy is a broad category that includes idiopathic disorders and toxic myocardial injury due to alcohol or certain drugs. Infiltrative myocardial lesions may accompany sarcoidosis, connective tissue disease, and other systemic conditions. Progressive muscular dystrophy and other neuromuscular disorders may involve the myocardium.

Table 30-1 lists EKG patterns found in cardiomyopathy patients. These abnormalities, alone or in combination, seldom lead directly to the diagnosis. As an exception, asymmetric septal hypertrophy may be identified in an appropriate clinical setting by exaggerated initial septal QRS forces, revealed by a tall R wave in V_1 and abnormal Q waves in the anterolateral leads or inferior leads. Cardiomyopathy is another cause of pseudoinfarction patterns. The EKG may at times be normal in patients with advanced cardiomyopathy.

Table 30-1 Principal EKG Abnormalities in Cardiomyopathy

Rhythm	PVCs, VT
	AF, AFl
	AV block
P waves	LAE
	RAE
QRS complexes	BBB
	Abnormal Q waves
	High voltage
	Low voltage
ST segment	Depressed
T waves	Inverted

Complete the following sentences:

1. In Figure 30-1, the PRI is _____ sec and _____ BBB is present, with QRS duration _____ -sec. Q waves are present in the _____ lead group.

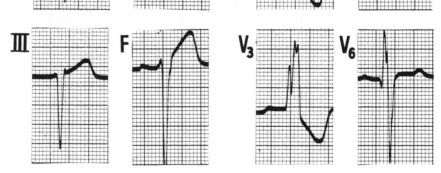

Figure 30-1

2. Figure 30-2, the EKG of a 42-year-old man with heart failure symptoms for 2 years, shows _____ BBB. P waves duration is _____ sec, consistent with _____ atrial enlargement.

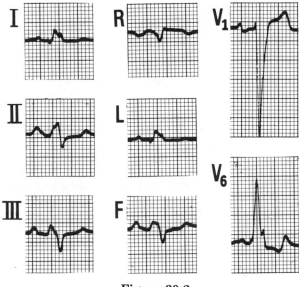

Figure 30-2

Review. The EKG manifestations of cardiomyopathy in Figure 30-1 include first degree AV block, with PRI 0.22 sec; RBBB, with QRS duration 0.16 sec; and a pseudoinfarction pattern, with Q waves in the anterolateral leads. In Figure 30-2, LBBB and LAE, with P wave duration 0.16 sec, are present in a patient with dilated cardiomyopathy.

Lesson 31

Hyperkalemia and Hypokalemia

In many clinical settings, EKG abnormalities are a valuable guide to cellular effects of abnormal serum potassium concentrations. Varying degrees of hyperkalemia and hypokalemia cause changes in ventricular repolarization, in conduction, and in impulse formation, as listed in Table 31-1.

Cardiac responses to abnormal serum K+ concentration depend in part on underlying disease, drug effects, and coexisting metabolic disorders. EKG findings accordingly do not have an entirely predictable relation to the degree of hyperkalemia or hypokalemia.

Figure 31-1(A) illustrates peaked T waves that suggest hyperkalemia, but could be normal. The T wave effects and increased QRS

Table 31-1 EKG Effects of Abnormal Serum Potassium Concentration

Serum [K$^+$] (meq/L)		EKG Effect
Hypokalemia	2 to 3	Large U wave
		Low T wave amplitude
	1 to 2.5	ST depression
Hyperkalemia	5 to 7	Tall, peaked T wave
	7 to 8	Wide QRS complex
	8 to 9	Low P wave
	9 to 10	Atrial arrest

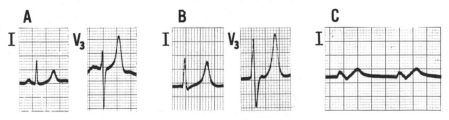

Figure 31-1 Effects of hyperkalemia of (A) mild, (B) moderate, and (C) severe degree.

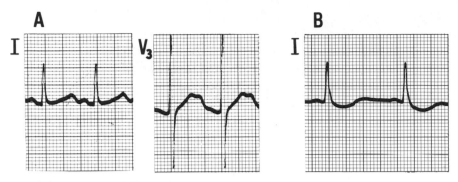

Figure 31-2 Effects of (A) moderate and (B) marked hypokalemia.

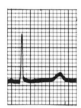

Figure 31-3 Prolonged QTI due to hypocalemia.

duration shown in Figure 31-1(B) are strong evidence that serum potassium level exceeds 7 meq/L. In Figure 31-1(C), atrial arrest and QRS width of 0.16 sec signal advanced hyperkalemia.

In lead I of Figure 31-2(A), large U waves due to hypokalemia nearly obscure the low T waves and give an impression of marked QTI prolongation. A simultaneous lead V_3 clearly separates the T wave and abnormal U wave. In Figure 31-2(B), more advanced hypokalemia has obliterated the T wave; U waves persist and sagging ST depression is present.

Hypocalcemia, in contrast to hypokalemia, causes true prolongation of the QTI. In Figure 31-3, T wave configuration is normal. QTI duration of 0.48 sec reflects ST segment prolongation due to hypocalcemia.

Complete the following sentence:

1. In Figure 31-4(A), EKG complexes obtained during treatment of diabetic ketoacidosis initially show _____ T waves consistent with _____ . In Figure 31-4(B), a later tracing shows _____ waves consistent with _____ .

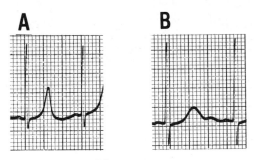

Figure 31-4

Review. Peaked T waves in Figure 31-4A correspond to a serum potassium concentration of 5.8 meq/L. Later, U waves are present and potassium concentration is 2.3 meq/L.

Lesson 32

Pericardial Disease

In Lessons 17 and 22, you learned that pericardial inflammation typically causes diffuse ST elevation without reciprocal changes. ST elevation resolves as inflammation subsides to be followed by T wave inversion, which may be the only EKG manifestation of chronic pericarditis. ST and T wave abnormalities due to pericardial hemorrhage resemble those of acute pericarditis. Large pericardial effusions, as found in

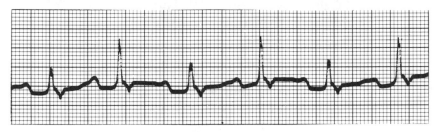

Figure 32-1 Electrical alternans as seen with large pericardial effusion.

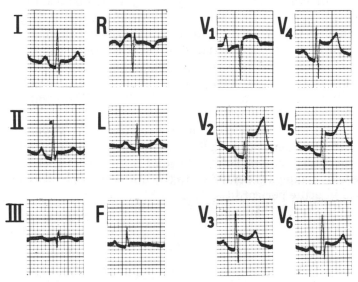

Figure 32-2 ST elevation due to pericardial hemorrhage.

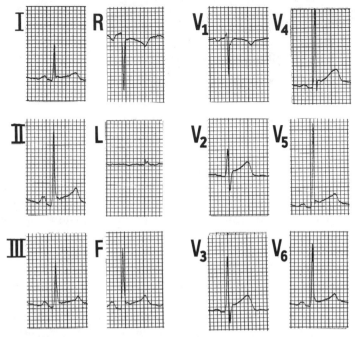

Figure 32-3   Acute pericarditis with generalized ST segment elevation and PR segment depression in limb leads.

chronic uremia or neoplastic involvement of the pericardium, may cause low QRS voltage. Large effusions may also be associated with the unusual phenomenon of electrical alternans illustrated in Figure 32-1. The change in QRS amplitude for alternate beats reflects a swinging cardiac motion within the pericardial sac. Electrical alternans rarely may occur in advanced cardiomyopathy.

Figure 32-2, the emergency room EKG of an 18-year-old patient treated for precordial stab wound, shows diffuse ST elevation due to pericardial hemorrhage.

Examine Figure 32-3, the admission EKG of a 28-year-old man with chest pain. Generalized ST segment elevation is present without reciprocal ST depression. Note that the PR segment between the P wave and the QRS complex is depressed in the limb leads, another abnormality found in acute pericarditis.

Lesson 33

Statistical Ideas in EKG Interpretation

Many pitfalls of 12-lead EKG interpretation can be avoided by attention to a simple principle: If a disease is unlikely to be present before a diagnostic test is performed, its presence will still be unlikely to some degree, regardless of a positive test, unless the test is completely reliable. This principle has applications throughout medical diagnosis. It will apply in some settings even to interpretation of histologic pathology, in spite of the high reliability of tissue examination. Abnormal EKG findings often increase the likelihood of a diagnosis without providing accurate confirmation, especially if the clinical setting is unknown. Lesson 33 will discuss several aspects of this principle:

Estimate of pretest likelihood.

Sensitivity and specificity of EKG findings.

Ways to express posttest likelihood.

One approach to estimating pretest likelihood of a diagnosis begins with the assumption that, in the absence of any information, all possible diagnoses are equally likely (Bayes' postulate). Every item of information, beginning simply with the patient's age and sex, changes the distribution of pretest probabilities.

Examine Figure 33-1. The patient is a 22-year-old man admitted to a Coronary Care Unit with ventricular tachycardia. Abnormal Q waves and T wave inversion in the anterolateral leads are consistent with anterolateral myocardial infarction, an unlikely diagnosis in this age group. Because of low pretest likelihood, the diagnosis of infarction should be avoided. An echocardiogram confirmed that hypertrophic cardiomyopathy was the explanation for the pseudoinfarction pattern in this patient.

Pretest likelihood may also be influenced by information obtained from a patient's previous EKG. Examine Figure 33-2. The patient is a 46-year-old woman. Delayed R wave progression in V_1 to V_3 is an abnormal finding that may be innocuous or important. Figure 33-3 shows an EKG for the same patient taken a year earlier, when evidence of anteroseptal myocardial infarction was present. The pretest likeli-

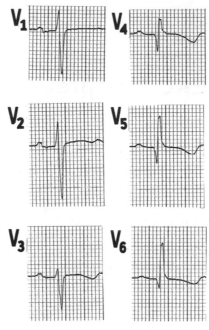

Figure 33-1 Pseudoinfarction pattern due to hypertrophic cardiomyopathy.

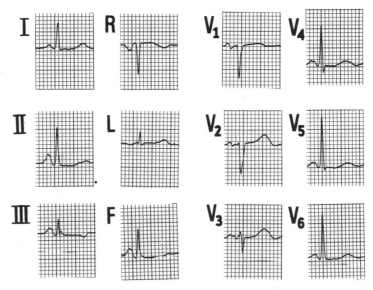

Figure 33-2 Delayed R wave progression.

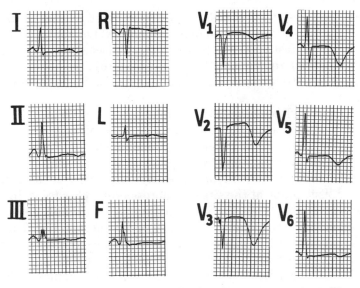

Figure 33-3 Anteroseptal myocardial infarction one year prior to Figure 33-2.

hood of this diagnosis for Figure 33-2 becomes 100%, and interpretation should state that minimal residual evidence of old anteroseptal infarction persists at this late stage of evolution of the infarction pattern.

Epidemiologic information has an especially important role in estimating pretest risk for CAD, particularly if a patient's coronary risk factors are known. This information must be used to interpret an abnormal exercise stress test when the patient is asymptomatic or has noncardiac chest pain. In a low risk group, especially for young women, horizontal ST depression at a high level of stress only slightly increases the risk that CAD is present.

Examine Figure 33-4. The patient is a 60-year-old woman with nearly constant chest tightness during a recent period of emotional stress. She has a normal blood pressure and serum cholesterol level. She does not smoke and has no family history of heart disease. She

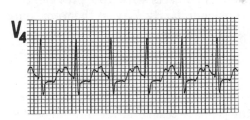

Figure 33-4 Abnormal ST segment depression.

stopped the stress test because of fatigue and had no chest pain. At an early stage of exercise, the test shows abnormal horizontal ST segment depression. Pretest risk of coronary artery disease for this patient is low. Posttest risk remains relatively low in spite of the abnormal result. A subsequent stress thallium scan showed no evidence of myocardial ischemia.

Extensive efforts have been made to determine the sensitivity and specificity of EKG abnormalities. Reliable determinations are difficult, however, in part because non-EKG criteria for the diagnosis under study may be elusive. For coronary artery disease, coronary arteriograms are often considered diagnostically definitive. But the severity of coronary obstruction at the site of atherosclerotic plaques is difficult to measure and, in addition, luminal diameter is not the only determinant of coronary flow. An ischemic response on an exercise test depends on other variables, such as extent of collateral flow beyond an obstruction.

Even if percentage values for diagnostic sensitivity and specificity of an EKG abnormality were precisely known, these values, unless they are 100%, would not completely determine the posttest risk of disease when the abnormality is present. A sensitive test is usually positive when the disease is present and a specific test is usually negative when the disease is not present, but neither of these variables relate to pretest risk, the prevalence of the disease in the population tested. A probability theorem, developed by the Rev. Thomas Bayes and published posthumously in 1763, provides a framework for considering these issues. According to this theorem, the posttest likelihood of disease when a test is positive can be defined as a function of sensitivity and specificity of the test, together with disease prevalence:

$$\text{Posttest probability } (+) = \frac{\text{sens} \times \text{prev}}{(\text{sens} \times \text{prev}) + (1 - \text{spec})(1 - \text{prev})}$$

In EKG interpretation, neither test sensitivity and specificity nor disease prevalence is precisely known. Consider, however, a set of hypothetical EKG criteria for the diagnosis of LVH and assume that these criteria are 90% sensitive and 90% specific. If applied in a health screening program of subjects with 10% prevalence of LVH, these criteria could be misleading. By Bayes' theorem, only 50% of positive diagnoses would be accurate:

$$\frac{(90 \times 10)}{(90 \times 10) + (10 \times 90)} = .5$$

In effect, the positive test removes the subject from the 10% prevalence group and places the subject in a 50% prevalence group. The test clearly does not establish a diagnosis in spite of high values for sensitivity and specificity.

Many common EKG findings must be interpreted with caution unless the pretest risk of a diagnosis is relatively high on the basis of available clinical information. High QRS voltage is sensitive, but not specific evidence for LV. Tall R waves in lead V_1 may be innocuous, but in appropriate clinical settings they may give strong evidence for RVH or for posterior wall myocardial infarction. Similarly, Q waves in leads III and aVF should not be considered diagnostic for inferior myocardial infarction unless the pretest risk is high.

It is clear, then, that EKG interpretation requires some method for expressing the likelihood of a diagnosis based in part on assumptions that are often subjective. Different interpreters may make different assumptions about the same EKG, depending in part on their experience and their willingness to accept risks of overdiagnosis or underdiagnosis. Especially when no clinical information is available, an interpreter may choose simply to describe the EKG findings. Alternatively, the interpreter may state a diagnosis modified by a term such as "probable" or "possible" as general indications of likelihood. Because other methods in cardiology have much greater reliability than the EKG for many important diseases, excessive reliance on EKG diagnosis is commonly unwise.

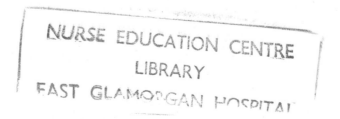

Glossary

The intent of a glossary, by dictionary definition, is "to render clear by comment." The terms chosen for discussion here are each a potential source of confusion. In some instances, traditional terms do not conform readily to current electrophysiologic concepts. Other terms have a variety of meanings that depend on their context. This glossary does not include items that receive detailed discussion in the text.

Arrhythmias—diagnostic terms: Advances in clinical and experimental electrophysiology have increasingly added to or modified established arrhythmia terminology. Arrhythmia classification and diagnostic terms generally refer to the chamber or structure in which the arrhythmia originates; the electrophysiologic mechanism, if known; and aspects of timing, such as prematurity, paroxysmal onset, or accelerated rate. Examples of current terminology for SVT and for AV block are given below. The use of a variety of synonyms for the same rhythm disorder is at times a source of confusion.

Atrioventricular block: Classification of AV block is most useful in terms that refer to the site of block, either in the AV node (proximal, type I) or in infranodal pathways (distal, type II). Older terms are less precise, especially for second degree AV block. Wenckebach first described the phenomenon of gradual AV conduction failure. Mobitz later labeled this phenomenon type I second degree AV block and defined type II, in which conduction fails abruptly. Four decades later, His bundle electrograms localized the anatomic site of these blocks respectively to the AV node and infranodal pathways. If eponyms are used, recommended terms for second degree AV block are type I (Wenckebach) and type II (Mobitz).

Atrioventricular dissociation: This term applies to a variety of rhythm disorders. Separate foci may control the atria and ventricles because of third degree AV block or because the atrial focus is slower than an independent ventricular focus, as during ventricular tachycardia without retrograde atrial activation, or during SB with junctional escape rhythm. When this term is used, the mechanism of dissociation should always be stated.

Automaticity: This important property of natural pacing fibers corresponds to cyclic spontaneous diastolic depolarization, phase 4 of the intracellular action potential, as illustrated for a typical SA node pacing fiber in Figure G-1. Rate of impulse formation in a pacing fiber depends on maximum membrane potential, on rate of phase 4 depolarization, and on the level of threshold potential for rapid depolarization (phase 0).

Axis: Linear axes are useful for describing the spatial orientation of EKG leads and of cardiac electrical forces. For each bipolar limb lead, a frontal plane linear axis connecting positive and negative electrodes is readily visualized. For unipolar limb leads, linear axes connect each electrode position, or positive pole, with a central zero point, and an extension of each axis indicates a negative direction, or pole, for the corresponding lead. Similarly, axes for unipolar chest leads connect each electrode position with a central zero point in the horizontal plane. A cardiac electrical force will have a spatial direction, or axis, that originates at the central zero point. An EKG wave will have an axis that corresponds to the axis of the cardiac electrical force it represents.

Bigeminy: A bigeminal rhythm exists whenever ventricular beats, or QRS complexes, occur in a series of pairs. Mechanisms for bigeminy include premature atrial or ventricular beats after every sinoatrial beat; AFl with alternating 2:1 and 4:1 AV conduction; 3:2 SA node exit block; and second degree AV block with 3:2 conduction. Although this term is most commonly used when premature beats are responsible for the paired ventricular rhythm, it is not a precise term and its mechanism should be stated.

Conduction: Spread of depolarization through the heart chambers follows a complex pattern. Specialized conduction fibers are comparable to superhighways surrounded by a dense network, or syncytium, of slower conduction paths through unspecialized contractile myocardial cells. Depolarization spreads from cell to cell in all available directions. Fibrous tissue barriers normally prevent spread of

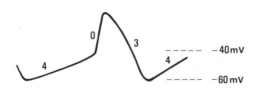

Figure G-1   Intracellular action potential for an automatic SA fiber with maximum diastolic potential −60 mV and threshold potential −40 mV.

depolarization from atria to ventricles except through the AV node-His bundle conduction pathway.

EKG complex: A complex, or group of closely related waves, may represent a complete cardiac cycle, a single event (QRS complex), or related events (ventricular complex of QRS, ST segment, and T wave).

EKG lead: This term may apply to an electrode or pair of electrodes, to an axis that defines the spatial orientation of an electrode or pair of electrodes, or to the complexes recorded by an electrode or pair of electrodes.

Electrical force: Cardiac electrical forces, although of low electrical power, measurably alter the body's internal electromagnetic field. At any instant of the cardiac cycle, the direction and magnitude of this alteration can be represented as a vector originating from a central source (or dipole). Cardiac electrical forces may be classified according to their anatomic source, their EKG manifestation, or their electrophysiologic mechanism—namely, atrial forces, QRS forces, and repolarization forces.

Electrical impulse: It is useful to refer to cell depolarization as an impulse, an electrical event that causes a response. In the heart, this response may be myofibrillar contraction or conduction to adjacent cells, or both together, depending on cell type.

Escape beat or rhythm: This term refers to normal activity of a natural secondary pacemaker when it captures cardiac contraction because normally dominant natural pacemakers have slowed excessively or have encountered a conduction block.

Hypertrophy and enlargement: For cardiac chambers, these terms are basically synonymous. EKG criteria do not reliably distinguish between chamber dilation and chamber wall thickening, anatomic findings that commonly coexist in association with increased chamber wall mass.

Internodal tracts: Anatomic pathways between the SA and AV nodes are much less distinct than the conduction bundles below the AV node. Their physiologic importance remains under debate. SA depolarization, however, does not spread through the atria in a random pattern. The concept of internodal tracts, although a simplification, is useful as applied to experimental and clinical observations concerning atrial activation and P wave configuration.

Normal: This term may have several connotations. In statistical use, it applies to a defined range of values, usually equal to two standard deviations above and below the mean value for a normal distribution. This application is seldom appropriate in EKG interpretation. In a broad sense, the term normally may apply to an unusual or atypical finding that is innocuous in an individual clinical context. Many normal values used in this text are based on those published by the New York Heart Association (*Nomenclature and Criteria for Diagnosis of Diseases of the Heart and Great Vessels,* 8th ed. Little, Brown, Boston, MA, 1979).

Supraventricular tachycardia: As generally applied, this term refers to any rhythm with ventricular rate greater than 100 bpm that originates above the bifurcation of the His bundle. When the mechanism of such a tachycardia is known, specific terms should be used. Paroxysmal SVT in adults is usually AV nodal reentrant tachycardia. In some instances, an AV bypass tract may be the basis for reentrant tachycardia that simulates a supraventricular mechanism, although its reentry circuit involves both atrial and ventricular pathways.

Index

Page numbers followed by f indicate figures; those followed by t indicate tables.

QRS complex(es) *(Continued)*
    and ventricular ectopic depo-
        larization, 77–82, 78f–79f,
        81f–82f
    and ventricular hypertrophy,
        83–87, 84f–86f
    relationship to ST segments, T
        waves, and QTI, 39–41,
        39f–41f
QTI. *See* QT interval
QT interval, 39, 39f, 41–43, 42f, 43f,
    43t
    and hypocalcemia, 192, 192f
    and PVCs, 146
Q wave abnormalities. *See also* QRS
        complex(es), abnormal
    and cardiomyopathy, 90, 90f
    and myocardial infarction, 89, 91,
        91f, 92f, 93
    and WPW syndrome, 90–91, 90f

RAD. *See* Right axis deviation
RAE. *See* Right atrial enlargement
RBB. *See* Right bundle branch
RBBB. *See* Right bundle branch
        block
Reciprocal changes, 21f, 22
Recording errors, 45–46, 46f
Reentry, and atrial tachyarrhyth-
        mia, 59–64, 59f
Repolarization, 7, 8t
Right atrial enlargement (RAE), and
        abnormal P waves, 66–68,
        67f, 182, 183f
Right axis deviation (RAD), of QRS,
        32–33, 32f, 182, 183f
    and RVH, 85, 86
Right bundle branch (RBB), location
        of, 4f, 5
Right bundle branch block (RBBB),
        182, 182f
    and abnormal QRS complex, 71,
        72–73, 72f, 73f

and PAC, 141, 141f
    and ST segment depression, 112,
        112f
Right ventricular hypertrophy
        (RVH), 178–182, 181t, 182f,
        183f
    and QRS abnormalities, 85–87,
        85f, 86f
    and ST segment depression, 111,
        111f
RVH. *See* Right ventricular hyper-
        trophy
R wave progression, 29–30, 29f, 30f

SA. *See* Sinoatrial *entries*
Sensitivity, of EKG findings,
        200–201
Sinoatrial (SA) exit block, 133–135,
        134f, 135f
Sinoatrial (SA) node
    functions of, 5–6, 9–10, 9f, 10f
    and junctional pacemaker, 53
    location of, 3–4, 4f
    and P wave measurement, 24–25
Specificity, of EKG findings, 200–201
Spontaneous electrical impulse for-
        mation, 5–6
Statistics, and EKG interpretation,
        197–201, 198f–200f
    posttest likelihood, 200
    pretest likelihood, 197–200
    sensitivity and specificity,
        200–201
Stress test, 106–107
ST segment, 8, 8f, 9, 39–41, 39f–41f
    abnormal
        depression. *See* ST segment
            depression
        elevation. *See* ST segment ele-
            vation
ST segment depression
    and AFl, 112, 112f
    from digitalis, 111, 111f